All Scripture references taken from KJV, unless otherwise indicated.

THE FAT DEMONS,

Breaking Demonic & Generational Curses

by Dr. Marlene Miles

Third printing.

First printing, 1999, Second printing 2000, Third printing, 2022.

ISBN: 978-1-960150-09-7

Paperback Version

Table of Contents

The FAT DEMONS

Breaking Demonic and Generational Curses

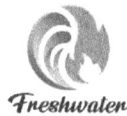

Freshwater Press, USA

The FAT of the Land

My dad is an Old Testament man who would read the Bible out loud for hours at a time. He no doubt read about the **fat** of the land. Daddy didn't have a Concordance or Hebrew-Greek dictionary, so as he read, he understood fat to mean fat. An old-fashioned Baptist, daddy didn't have the concordance of the Holy Spirit either, so he understood fat to mean fat. At mealtime, Daddy's plates were fuller than anyone's. Mom is an excellent cook, but it was as though Daddy was trying to <u>eat</u> the *fat* of the land that he read about in the Scriptures. We'd ask Daddy, *Don't you think you're getting big?*

He would reply, adjusting his pants back above his dunlap. *"I'm prosperous."*

Now that we've read the Bible for ourselves, we understand more. Dad was brought up during the Great Depression and was taught to eat **all** of his food when he *had* food. That clean your plate mentality carried over to adulthood, and when he added his experiences to what he read in the Bible, it became a confirmation for Daddy to <u>eat</u>. Being fat in the old days was a sign of prosperity while being thin was a sign of poverty. Considering the dearth of food during the Depression and believing that *fat* meant prosperous, Daddy ate abundantly to prove that he was no longer poor.

Fat still means fat, but now we have Hebrew-Greek dictionaries, concordances, and revelation through the Holy Spirit, to help us understand the different kinds of Old Testament fat. There was the fat of animals, the fat of man, and the fat of the land. The fat of the land is the prosperity or abundance, spoils, resources, and harvest of the actual land. When God says we can *eat the fat*, He means partake of or use the resources of the land.

Almost all of the Old Testament fat is metaphorical, not literal. God is not saying to eat fat and get physically heavy.

And take your father and your households, and come unto me, and I will give you the good of the land of Egypt. And he shall eat the fat of the land.

Genesis 45:18

The Sacrifice of Fat

While there is much talk about fat in the Old Testament, the word, *fat* is not even in the New Testament. Could it be that with the birth of Jesus *fat* became obsolete? Oh, were at so. But in a sense, it is true. The sacrifice of animals was practically an everyday thing for Old Testament people, but things changed drastically by the time of the New Testament. Animal sacrifice was common under the Old Covenant, so God told man exactly how to handle the meat, blood, and fat of that ritual.

> And the priest shall burn them upon the altar. It is the food of the offering made by fire for a sweet savor. All the fat is the Lord's. It shall be a perpetual statute. For your generations, throughout all your dwellings, that ye eat neither fat nor blood. Leviticus 3:16-17

The eating of the sacrificial fat was as abominable as eating the blood. Life was in the blood, therefore ingesting it was forbidden. The fat was a delicacy; it was the Lord's and not to be eaten. Eating marbled steaks or roast that had fat in them was fine if they were prepared for food. But the *suet,* the fat (*suet*) of the sacrificed animal was entirely the Lord's. To eat the Lord's portion of a sacrifice was a religious violation punishable swiftly and severely.

Speak to the children of Israel saying, you shall eat no manner of fat, or ox or sheep, or of goat. Leviticus 7:23

If the animal was not killed, but died on its own, then no part of it should be eaten.

And the fat of the beast that dieth of itself, and the fat of that which is torn with beasts, may be used in any other use, but ye shall in no wise eat of it. Leviticus 7:24

The Bible has everything, even the rules for roadkill.

There may not be any talk of fat in the New Testament because the animal sacrifice became obsolete by the once and for all sacrifice of the Lamb of God, Jesus Christ.

But this man, after he had offered one sacrifice for sins forever, sat down on the right hand of God. Hebrews 10:12

8

Thank God that in the Better Covenant, there are no more animal sacrifices. But does that mean we should eat as much of anything as we want? No, you'd never see an all you can eat sign at an Old Testament sacrificial service or Holy Communion. Those are designed to give God honor.

How can we, stop overeating, especially on feast holidays and honor God? Here's how: The Old Testament sacrifice of fat doesn't have to be an old sacrifice anymore. Just as we offer the sacrifice of praise or the sacrifice of our offerings. Why not offer God the sacrifice of fat? Eating no meat or dairy products would be a true sacrifice. Offer Him the delicacy; offer God the best.

The sacrifice of fat: Fast fat for a week or a month and see how it pleases God and blesses you.

*Consult your own physician before beginning any diet or exercise program. Some fatty acids are essential for good health. A long term fast that reduces fat instead of eliminating fat completely can also be very beneficial.

The Fat of The Man

The murder of Eglon, the king of Moab, was the first talk of physical fat in the Bible. Eglon's fat was so profuse that when he was stabbed, the dagger that was thrust in him stuck. Why we are told this story is left to your interpretation, but that's a lot of fat.

... And Eglon was a very fat man. Ehud... Took the dagger.... And thrust it into his belly. And the haft also went in after the blade, and the fat closed upon the blade so that he could not draw the dagger out of his belly.... Judges 3:17, 22-23

The Bible warns of overeating and lustful appetites. Eglon may have had a hedonistic appetite. This was a worldly king who oppressed Israel and gave in to his own lusts. On the opposite end is Eli. The priest, Eli was a man of God, but he also ate to become a very heavy man. **Food does not discriminate, so the man must.** It does not matter if you are in the world or saved, overeating will add fat. Proverbs 23:2 warns that the man that eats too much should take a knife to his own throat. Eli's death didn't involve a knife; he heard word of what had happened to the Ark of the Covenant and died in a fall. God's judgments are spiritual. They don't necessarily have to do with a person's size or weight.

> ... He fell from off the seat backward by the side of the gate, and his neck break, and he died, for he was an old man and heavy. 1 Samuel 4:18

(Is this where the term, *keeled over dead* comes from?)

Possibly if Eli hadn't been so big, his fall, though a response to a spiritual matter may not have been fatal. Eating a lot doesn't prove prosperity, help agility, or increase lifespan. And if the why and how of eating is not understood food may be a route for demonic entrance, footholds, traps, or snares. Fatal or non-fatal falls can result in the spiritual or physical realm from food and misuse of it. Food can be the cause of addictions and death.

The root of many people's troubles, problems, and curses is **food**. An obedient Adam and Eve in the garden would not have eaten of the Tree, but while under the temptation of the actual devil, if they had fasted neither would have fallen into sin.

When Jesus was in the Wilderness for 40 days and nights, He was personally tempted of the devil like Adam and Eve, except Jesus won. Jesus was fasting. Was that a coincidence? No. God's Kingdom doesn't work by accident or chance. Jesus did not stumble on or happen into His ministry. Jesus did not

11

happen to be fasting at the time He was tempted. He was showing us how to overcome even in times of temptation.

The first part of Jesus's temptation was the offer of **food**. Why would the devil offer food unless there was something to it? Why do you bless food before eating? Is there something in food, about food, or about eating food that needs to be *blessed* before consumption? Probably. When asking grace, you thank God, and you ask that the food is both nourishing and safe to eat. You mean physically safe, hoping that the food will not make you sick or kill you. We should add **spiritually** safe in our prayers; if we consider the spiritual, as we should, we wouldn't eat a lot of things that we eat.

Food is spiritual?

Yes, it can be. You're spiritual so what goes into your body must be considered seriously. Why do you pray over what you eat? And if your physical body is being used for spiritual works, godly works, then what you put in it, how you treat it, is very important. When you care about something, and you want it to last a long time, you take care of it. You need a physical body to exert your authority in the Earth, that is, you need a physical body to exert yourself spiritually. To exert yourself effectively, you need a healthy and fit body. Dead men don't sing, and sick men aren't as effective in ministry as healthy men, so you must take care of your body.

Food gives natural strength, as in Popeye's power spinach rush. Our God confounds the wise--, how does a fasting man have **more** spiritual strength than a man who eats? If Jesus had eaten in that first Temptation, He would have been spiritually weakened rather than strong, thank God He didn't.

Am I saying the spiritually weak overeat? If food is a temptation to you and you overeat, then you are weak. When giving in to one temptation, the next temptation could easily overtake a person. After eating everything on the table, eating the pie or cake is as easy as pie. Or cake.

If you are under temptation or feel you're about to enter temptation, consider fasting.

Party Over Here

An old TV ad claims you can make friends with Kool-Aid. Food and beverage often accompany social events. Sometimes the food *is* the entertainment. When believing to be among friends, guards are let down. Consider how the prophets eating at Jezebel's table, (1 Kings 18:19) did her bidding. Many business deals are made over meals. Mafia movies depict bad things happening in restaurants as the victims dine. When it comes to attack, ambush and deception, eating is one of the ultimate distractions.

When planning a party, which is made first, the menu or the guest list? Depends on what you want to accomplish, *right*?

Many parties start with food, then escalate to alcohol or drugs. If you told someone you were having a drug party, who would come? OK, I asked that. One enemy trick is to bring out alcohol and drugs after the party crowd has gathered. Luke 15:23 invites the eating of food and the making of merry, which is to *party*. That passage in Luke was about something good, combined with something bad. Food with drugs for example--, an old Devil trick is exposed. A spoonful of sugar helps the medicine go down. The food is sugar, something you know and like, but the deception is when the medicine is not really medicine.

Food is necessary for life. Thankfully, God has promised us all things that pertain to life and godliness,
(2 Peter 1:3) and He provides an abundance in our culture. We have the luxury of eating three or more meals a day. These can be times of temptation if something bad is tied to the activity, if the eating is done improperly, is mishandled, or deception is slipped in. Free food can be *found* at happy hours where alcoholic beverages are sold. Food abounds at gambling events, and extremely cheap food is known to be at casinos. Food courts are in the mall. You are encouraged to stay all day, use up all your free time, and overspend. Besides having the luxury of regular meals, we are bombarded with food temptations almost everywhere we go.

I recently saw fresh popcorn vending at a courts building as if court is entertainment. Complete food courts and state municipal courts buildings are sure to be next, (I'm prophesying). There's a large, large crowd of people. They can't leave until their numbers are called. They are stressed out, nervous, and worried--, all the conditions under which many eat. Most left home in a hurry without eating. Food courts, even in such an odd place, carries a big potential for making money. Don't be surprised when you see it come to pass.

Talk about a party! Sodom and Gomorrah, which is well known for sex perversions had more food than many may have realized. Don't joke that when certain kinds of men get together, they cook and decorate. It's no joking matter. The *spirit of sexual perversion*, besides what we know it can do, really influences--, eating. Other than eating, there may be nothing innocent about this bold and perverse *spirit*. This *spirit*, like too many others, influences man to the lust of the flesh, and to live life to the fullest, whatever the that *fullest* may be.

Fulfilling an exaggerated lust for food on a large scale has often been the indication of the beginning of the end of many civilizations. Our society is exhibiting characteristics similar to the declining Roman Empire, which had just about every flesh desire. Polygamy, concubines and harems were legal. Men had as many women as they wanted, but they wanted more, different, strange, and perverted. They even built homosexual bath houses. Fulfilling the lust for food and flesh pleasures, they hosted feast banquets and orgies that lasted days on end. They ate while reclining as the Empire was declining.

Christians were publicly fed to lions where gladiators fought them to the death. **Christians were not in style.** They *were* the entertainment, being sacrificed regularly before the time of Emperor Constantine.

Where there is entertainment, there is food. Count on it. If you see food, no matter what's going on the people believe that what they are doing is:

- OK, acceptable, or all right.

- Entertainment, no matter how wrong it is.

To a Roman, a barbarian didn't know Greek philosophy and what implement to use at the dining table. The world still judges by the outward. Avid Christians are still considered fanatics. You can see how the world we live in is very much the same--, it is about parties, wild sex, and giving in to the flesh. It is all about now and today; most people are not thinking about Eternity. Unfortunately, the worldly man is *still* only looking at the outward and he still wants the same things as ever, food, sex, parties, fun, prosperity, creature comforts and flesh desires.

Like Jesus, we disciples must still witness to the unsaved no matter what their spiritual flaws, sinful desires, lack, of communication or level of understanding may be.

Because the things of God are spiritually understood and the world does not have God's Spirit, communication may be strained, or understanding may be lacking between the saved and the unsaved. We Christians must still practice our faith and witness to others; it's the Great Commission, (Acts 1:8). We

17

cannot fail to share the Gospel with others. Don't give up on people. Not even those with the hardest of hearts. Remember there was a time when you didn't have God's Spirit. You may not have been a murderer or a hater, but maybe you were. But look at how far you've come because of God's love and Grace.

Because of God's Spirit, your understanding has been opened, (Ephesians 1:18). You are, and are becoming, more spiritually aware and alert to deception. Caution: Food can still be one such deception. To date, many books have been written about foods as aphrodisiacs. Reporting that food can get you sex, wining and dining. Certain foods such as oysters are said to enhance sexual enjoyment. If this is true, then has food been used on you as an aphrodisiac or as a tool to lull you into a false sense of comfort?

Women are taught as girls that the way to a man's heart is through his stomach. After eating, blood flows to the stomach. As digestion begins, sleepiness, or extreme relaxation may follow. Awareness decreases, and laziness may increase. One may be more prone to suggestion. (*Why don't we get married?* or more easily influenced? *(Honey, I want a new car.)*

You may be fed so you can then be LED. *Let's go to the mall.* If you fed a dog or a cat, it will follow you almost anywhere. You've heard it said, there is no free lunch; are you being *fed* for this reason? Something happens when folks are fed. Guards are let down, loyalties are formed, and deals are made. The devil knows this. Careful, in the world everyone who feeds you may not be a friend.

> Are you being fed,
> so you can be led?

That does not mean don't eat with people, nor does it mean don't accept invitations that involve food. It does not mean that people perceive your invitations in a negative way, necessarily. That only means in any situation, use Wisdom and discernment. Don't let food and the offer of food deceive you into thinking that everything is OK. Go with your *first mind*. If you think they want something from you, be prayerful that you choose to bless them or give them what they want rather than being taken advantage of; but go ahead and enjoy your meal.

On a scarier note, in some cultures food and beverage are used as the vehicle for pagan curses, but the greater one is in you. Still consider the sources of your food blessings and don't forget to ask God's grace over your meals. Remember to not only pray that your food is physically and *spiritually* safe to consume.

Prayers

19

I bind *whoredoms*, sex sins, lust and perversions, especially sins brought on by food. I cast them out in the Name of Jesus. I *loose* the Holy Spirit, holiness and temperance in my life. I'm aware, alert and ask God for spiritual discernment, so I am not deceived by anything. In the Name of Jesus, Amen.

Food is not entertainment.

A Hill of Beans

Esau traded his birthright for a hill of beans, I mean bean soup. He was so hungry, he swapped his blessings for food, (Genesis 25:30-33). Jacob fed his brother, Esau and then led him down the path of deception. You'd never do that, would you? It's never been done to you, has it? You would never trade your birthright of salvation and eternal life, for food, drink, good times, or fleshly desires, would you? You wouldn't be willing to trade eternal salvation for eternal hell, so you can party and do what you want, while on this temporary flesh journey through Earth, would you?

That's what the devil wants to know. That's what the devil keeps asking, every time he offers you something. Will you trade your God-stuff, your gifts, your Salvation, your promises and blessings for food? Is food all it takes? The devil will get that for you. Or will you trade it for sex? How about perverted sex?

Does it take that, because he can get that for you, too. Will you trade it for murder? What is it for which you will trade your Salvation and your reward? Will you trade it for money, or fame? *What do you want?*

There are no promises or warnings about the consequences of what you want. The devil doesn't care about you, even though you may think he's getting you something to make you *happy*. He's a corrupt businessman, who is saying, *"What do you want? What will you accept in trade to give me the thing(s) I want from you?"* Deceptively the devil looks like he's in the business to get something for you, but he's really trying to take something from you. Satan would steal your soul, (mind, intellect, and emotions), but he can't if you are saved and walking upright in the LORD. The only way he can get it, or any part of it is if you give it willingly, or if you sin, don't repent, and it is taken legally. Trading is legal. Deception is legal. If you accept something from the devil, then you have to give up what you promised him, or the known cost of that trade. The devil wants you to trade your God-stuff for whatever he's offering. And with that trade, barter, or theft, comes pain, torture and torment—either now, and/or later, in hell.

The purpose of Jesus' Wilderness temptation was to show the reality and the gravity of the temptations that man may face and model the proper responses. Jesus had just gotten all of His credentials; He had just received the highest anointing: the Christ anointing. He was graced with full power, yet no man knew it yet. (the

> The devil's ultimate goal is to affect your soul's eternal address; he wants you in hell with him.

devil comes early and often.) Satan came offering worldly gifts; things to try to trade Jesus for what God had just given Him. What is the first thing the devil thought could tempt Jesus? **Food**.

The devil doesn't care, he will come for your gifts before they are even used, as he tried with Jesus. Many times, he comes before the gifts are received or even known about. This is why it is crucial for children and teens to be taught, trained, and nurtured spiritually. Their lives need to be spoken in to, so they know who they are, and what their gifts and talents are, at the earliest age possible.

Let's Make a Deal was a game where people traded what they had, what they thought they had, or what they thought they were going to get for things seen and unseen. That's what the devil wants you to do, like Esau, when he was hungry--, make a deal. And that's what worldliness is all about --, to distract, tempt and take way the gifts of God before they are used or even realized. The devil may even make people aware that they have certain gifts; put a false value on them, then enslave them for his purposes. For example, people may take certain God-given gifts and pervert them for personal financial gain. If the gifted person is made aware of their godly gifts, educated, trained, taught, is in proper relationship with God and in proper fellowship with the saints, then they won't trade or be tricked out of priceless God-given gifts.

Not to mention the prayer covering they'd be under because of being under authority, and in right relationship. If Esau had fully realized what his birthright was, he probably would not have traded it for food. And, if you recall the story, Esau was out in the wilderness alone, hunting. He was not in fellowship, but Jacob was connected to the family. Take a lesson here.

You Don't Have Anything to Lose

The *"You don't have anything to lose"* lie has surely been presented to you. *"Go ahead, try it, do it, you don't have anything to lose."* You may not look like you have anything to lose; you may not even feel that you have anything to live for. You may not feel special, or set aside, or even know your purpose yet, but if God made you, you've got something of great value. And if the devil is pursuing you, that confirms it. You are and have tremendous value. But what you have is not of value unless you:

- Know what you have.

- Know that it has value. And.

- You know how to use it.

When someone asks you what do you have to lose, you need to know that you have great gifts and abundance from God, but He didn't give it to you to lose it. Usually, the person asking the question is in the world and can't recognize the God things about you anyway. Don't take advice, counsel, or direction from the ungodly, (Psalms 1:1). You have a lot, but it's not to lose. And it's not for losing. It's for winning.

Declarations

My Salvation is more important to me than anything anyone could offer me, especially the devil. I refuse and reject temptations, whether it is simply food or other obvious violations against God's commandments. My soul's eternal address is with God, and my soul will arrive safely intact and to the glory of God. God has given me many gifts, talents, and abilities.

I do not have anything that I'm willing to lose.

I am victorious in Christ. I am not made for losing.

In Jesus' Name, Amen.

Fattened Up for The Kill

(Sacrifice)

Hansel and Gretel, of storybook fame, wandered into hostile witch territory. The witch, cannibalistic and slight of sight, perceived by their bony wrists that they were not fat enough to eat. So she set out to fatten them up. That is exactly what we do to the Thanksgiving goose and then sing songs about it. The fatted calf was prepared for the once Prodigal Son, (Luke 15:23). The fattened turkey looks better on the platter and is considered to taste better. Bigger is better; it's the American way. Americans really like that, the very thing that was set aside for God.

Fat.

The witch offered Hansel and Gretel everything they liked, and they ate. There would have been no strategy in offering things that they wouldn't eat. Devilish temptations are always things you like. To entice a person into a sex sin, the devil will send someone attractive. To entice an eating sin, food that you really enjoy will be made available to you, especially if you've declared a fast.

When fattened up, the witch was ready to consume them. Just like the witch, after being baited with the things you desire, the devil begins the switch to spring a trap. Satan offers things you like for a reason, and it's not because he likes you.

Or the devil, even if he has access to you because of your lifestyle and choices, may leave you alone, allowing you to feel secure and comfortable for a while. You may think that your success is because of your own hard work. You may be working hard, but if you're not worshipping and serving God, the devil may sit back and let you think you're living the perfect life, (for a time). Satan won't place many obstacles, if any if you're not serving God. If he did, then you might become distraught and seek God. Why would the devil want you to do that? If you're not saved and serving God, you're going to hell anyway so the devil can spend his energy trying to wreak havoc on the lives of other people.

When you're comfortable, you'll be thinking, *That can't happen to me,* or *I've got it made so I can do whatever I want and there's no consequence.* That's the physical and mental comfort the devil wants you to trust in. Watch out!
Maybe you're also thinking:

- I don't need to go to church.

- I don't need to live in holiness as long as I do my sinning out of town where no one knows me.

- If I'm selective with whom I sin, they won't tell and I won't tell, it'll be OK.

- I don't need to read the Bible. I don't need to pass or pray. That's for sinners, heathens and poor people.

The bait has been offered and taken, but the devil may be doing nothing right now but watching you sink deeper and deeper in sin. **Sin, without immediate consequence makes the Sinner believe falsely that there are no consequences.** Now that you're deceived into being spiritually comfortable, you believe that you don't need to change anything about yourself; you're perfect and you've got life all figured out. The reality is you've done so much wrong stuff, but nothing has happened--, so you think nothing is going to happen. You are **fat** in your comforts. And you're very wrong.

Listen closely--, do you hear the devil singing a song about a fat goose? It's fat now. It'll look much nicer on the platter. Now that it's fat, it will embarrass God more. Just when you don't think anything's going to happen that's when the devil tries to reel in the goose he's caught. You!

Fatter is more attractive, better tasting, better looking to the predator who might want you fat in your spiritual comforts, your natural abundance, or even physically fat? Who's after you? The devil. Who might want you heavier than you should be, slower

27

moving, weaker, not toned, out of condition, not able to run physically or spiritually? The devil wants you fattened up for the kill.

A lot of Pentecostals say they are *running for their lives*. They mean physical running. By running, I believe God means to work as a machine works. When a car motor *runs*, it's doing the thing it's supposed to do. You're supposed to *run* your course to the finish, (Acts 20:24). Running means doing what you have been called and anointed to do.

Thinking of marathon runners, thank God we don't have to physically run *from* the devil. And it's a good thing because how many *could*?

Spiritual fitness, (spiritual prosperity) means your prayers are instant and without ceasing. You are thankful to God. You study the Bible. You praise and worship. You also are faithful in church, paying tithes and giving offerings. Your spiritual machinery is working and ready to use at a moment's notice. Your gifts are stirred up and you are in the full armor of God, and ready with spiritual warfare if necessary. That's **running**.

Consumed In Fat

The Bible talks about being consumed in one's fat. Not like the dagger stuck in Eglon, but God says that when we have success, prosperity, and abundance, we get fat in our comforts and forget Him. That's what He calls consumed in our fat. God hates it when we are consumed in our own life goals and successes to His exclusion and what He has called us to do. God says we turn away from Him when we get **fat**.

Remember when you didn't have a car? Weren't you in great or better physical shape then? Now that you have creature comforts such as a house, job, and a nice vehicle, don't those luxuries make you fuller around the waist? It's human nature to forget what got you there. That's the *nature* that God is talking about when we get comfortable. Even physically when you were on your way up, you exercised and took care of yourself. Now that you have this nice position at the office, the gym is not even on your schedule. What have you taken off your *spiritual* schedule now that you think you don't have to ask God to bless your efforts anymore?

Being consumed in fat doesn't mean that heavy people don't serve God; some all the more. I am not saying that rich people don't serve God. The *comfortable* people are the ones who are **not** serving God, but they *think* they have everything they *think* they want. Those people believe that God is for the needy or the poor. They may believe that God is for who they were, and where they *used to be*. But every heavy person isn't comfortable any more than every thin person is. The temptation is that when everything is going fine in life to put God on a back burner for later usage. If you have a problem or a need, you can call on God. He can't be put on hold. Why? **Because God is the one who is really doing the calling, and when the person who is calling hangs up, the line goes dead.** By Mercy and Grace, He allows time for repentance and correction, but it will not always be this way.

> **But Jeshurun waxed fat and kicked. Thou art waxen fat, thou art grown thick. Thou art covered with fatness. Then he forsook God, which made him and lightly esteemed the rock of his salvation. Deut 32:15**

If you only *lightly* esteem God, He will lightly esteem you. Whether you are in your comforts or not, the way you treat God will be returned to you. Don't you have friends or relatives who only call or knock on your door when they want something? Do you think God is happy to see you only when you have a problem? Where is His praise, worship, and service when things are well with you?

When you're sending up a prayer, God may look down and see that *it's only you*. He sees the trouble you're in, He understands. He has compassion, but you're the one who comes to church sometimes, the one who pays the tithe sometimes and never gives offerings. You're the one who remains silent and seated during praise and worship. Don't be offended, but if you've only lightly esteemed God, you may have offended Him. Repent and rectify the problem now.

You've got to praise God because when you open your mouth and praise Him, you **highly** esteem Him. When you pay your tithes and give offerings, you highly esteem God. When you study and obey the Word, you highly esteem God. When you witness and minister to others, you highly esteem Him.

But if you're a silent saint, He may be thinking, **Oh, it's the one who lightly esteems me. I'll get to their prayer when I get to it, I will attend to the prayers of the righteous man and faithful first**. God has responsibility to bless those in His family first, just as you bless your own children first, and foremost. God knows that if He blesses you every time you have a problem and you're **not** serving Him, that you will never truly serve Him, even though you may say, "*God, if you bless me this time, if you get me out of this, I promise to come to church regularly. I*

promise to tithe. I promise this and I promise that."
God knows you won't. How does He know?

Because you haven't. He's gotten you out of stuff before, hasn't He? You've been seeing Him as a spiritual vending machine. You don't praise or worship or give offerings to a vending machine. You only go to it when you want something out of it. You must not lightly esteem God.

Develop a relationship with Him. He's a friend that sticks closer than a brother, (Proverbs 18:24).

Prayers

I esteem God, the Rock of my Salvation. I praise Him.

I repent of ever lightly esteeming God, and I purpose to serve Him with my whole self, whether times are FAT and comfortable or not.

I will not become FAT in comforts, but I will remember the Lord God who gives me power to get wealth.

As the Lord prospers me spiritually, I will not fail to serve, worship, praise, attend church, pray, study, share with others, minister, and be a blessing.

I endeavor to be spiritually fit, not spiritually FAT.

I will highly esteem the Rock of my Salvation.

I will praise the Lord. In the Name of Jesus, Amen.

Spiritually Fat

Spiritually FAT does not describe physical size.

There are all kinds of spiritually FAT people, and they are of all sizes. It describes several kinds of people. First, those who sit on the church pews not only every Sunday but also every service. They are there because they're *supposed* to be. These spiritually FAT, are not holding the Pew down, they are not bearing the Spirit up necessarily--, they are just there.

They are the kind of people who believe that the first person who applies for a job should get it. They think the ideal person for a position at an office is the one who came first. They mistakenly believe that the employer is only looking for a warm body to fill the position. God has no responsibility to bless you because you are physically at church, any more than you get the job just because you came to the interview. You've got to bring your mind, experience and skills to that job, and they might need to match the needs of the employer and you've got to bring your mind, body and soul to church and be there in spirit and in truth, (John 4:23). *Being* at church because of fear of God, fear of hell, fear of falling into sin is just the start. (God doesn't want a relationship simply based on fear.) Some church regulars are as baby Christians who don't trust themselves out of the

33

pastor's sight. They are at church because they are *supposed* to be there, not because of the relationship with God. (Not yet, but prayerfully right relationship with God is growing.)

Some baby Christians may have even been drawing on the pastor's teachings for years or decades. They soak up the Word expressionless or with great emotion, waving hands in excitement, shouting, *Amen*! These appear to have their spiritual life together, but at the end of worship they put on their outside faces to go back to work or home, business as usual. Never a word, prayer or any ministry flows through them. They collect the Word for years, but do nothing with it, thereby staying baby Christians, (Hebrews 5:12).

God requires regular church attendance, (Hebrews 10:25). In addition, reading Christian books and listening to study sermons and lessons will enhance their knowledge of the Word. But collecting all manner of godly spiritual information, never using it, is like putting an expensive hand knit cashmere sweater and a cedar chest and saving it for a special occasion.

Your life here on Earth is a special occasion.

It's why you're here.

34

The Word of God is for this special occasion, that's why God provided it. Most pastors don't preach Heaven anymore; the Word you are hearing is for now. It's for applying to your daily, real life. Rhema is Living Word and that is for you right now.

If you don't know what to do with the Word or how to use it, pray for Wisdom and understanding. Ask for the Holy Spirit so you can rightly divide the Word, (2 Timothy 2:15). Once you divide the Word, it's like eating. Now you can take bites of it. You can take as much as you need when you need it. Spiritual food for spiritual fitness.

But, if you know what to do with the Word, and you are among those who only harbor spiritual knowledge to use at church fellowships, that's another story. The choir already knows what you know. Why not take the Word out to your workplace, your home, your community, and bless those who haven't heard the Good News of the Gospel? Being spiritually miserly is a **FAT Demon**. It can make you *spiritually* fat.

Declarations

I receive and use spiritual food properly.

I reject spiritual fat. I share and minister spiritual food to others as God leads. I reject a miserly spirit.

Fat In Revelation Knowledge

Praise God, you are past the place where you only *collect* spiritual information. Perhaps you have been witnessing or ministering in the grocery stores and highways and byways. You might even talk to people where you work or at the bus stop. You may talk to people who may not be saved. Praise God. Maybe you are faithful in attending church, faithful in paying tithes and giving offerings. Faithful in studying the Bible, and faithful in ministry. Since God has been able to trust you with the little things in life, He may be now trusting you with revelation. God may be revealing new and wonderful things to your heart that you've never heard anywhere before--, things that set you on fire or make your heart soar. What are you doing with it? If nothing, then you are spiritually fat on revelation knowledge.

Perhaps you've written it all down in a book, a journal, or a manuscript. Do you have a collection of poems, short stories, or sermons that the Lord has given you, Wisdom that the Lord may have awakened you in the middle of the night to impart? Have you shared any of those things with anyone as God has led? Perhaps you've been faithful to record the new melody you woke up singing, and perhaps He gave you the anointed words as well. Is that song published, recorded, or even shared with the Music ministry of your Church? That song could heal, deliver, or uplift someone. You may not know who, but God knows. Revelation **FAT** is a terrible thing.

Are you wondering why your ministry isn't taking off? God's not holding you back. You are to minister what God has already given you. Like Samuel to Eli, a person's ministry often begins with a service to another ministry first. Be faithful to your church and leaders. Then God can bless you.

Thank God you are talking to others, and it's great to share of what you've received from man and from God through revelation. If you are not yet receiving, keep the faith. When you speak to or witness to someone out of your own relationship with God, you are much more effective than just repeating what the pastor said on Sunday. What the pastor said was for you. Some of it may be for that sinner you're witnessing to, but God gives fresh manna from Heaven for each occasion. Share, don't covet revelation. The miserly covetous spirit that won't share revelation is a **FAT Demon**.

A saved friend loves to call and talk about the

Word. We share the Lord's bright light being turned on in our hearts and minds, even though neither of us had a pulpit. We shared by telephone, e-mail, cards, letters, and notes by any means that we could. We shared with others, even if it was only one person at a time. We *ministered* the Good News of Jesus and the revelation we received by the Holy Spirit; you can do that too. **That is ministry.**

There are some *spiritually* fat who receive revelation and keep it hidden. I'm not talking about Mary who couldn't disclose information about the conception of Jesus. Neither am I talking about information that the Lord has instructed you **not** to share yet. Many times, He gave the Prophet a word and told him, **"Not yet."** John the Divine ate the words read from the Little Book, (Revelations 10:9) because it was not the time to share it yet. I'm talking about sharing a word in season and you know, in your knower it's a word in season. Your heart may be pounding, your pulse may be racing, you are so excited, but fear may have gripped you. Fear will cause you to sit on that Pew when God is saying get up. Fear can make you spiritually FAT. The *spirit of fear* is a **FAT Demon.**

If you are waiting for someone to "release" you into ministry, pray to God and see if the Holy Spirit will release you, if all the leaders you've met seem to be telling you don't and no, rather than go ahead.

Prayers & Declarations

I receive and use spiritual food properly.

I reject spiritual fat. I receive and share revelation as the Lord directs. I do not harbor it.

I bind up and cast out the *spirit of fear* in my life. And I *loose* the Spirit of love, power and a sound mind, in the Name of Jesus.

Fat In Gifts and Talents

There are many who are fat in gifts and talents. I call that gift or talent fat. Some can sing like a songbird, play an instrument, or build a bookshelf masterfully, but they still sit on the pew. You've been a member of your church for five years, you've been in fellowship after fellowship, and you have God-given abilities, talents, and skills, but no one knows. This is also spiritual fat. Is it fear or selfishness that keeps you seated and keeps you from sharing? You've got yours, your salvation and your spiritual gifts, your house and car. Do you care about anybody else?

Bob majored in photography in college but worked in another field. No one in his church knew. The church's video minister moved out of state suddenly, but Bob told no one in of his video and photography skills because he didn't want to have to come to church all day and tape. The *spirit of selfishness* is a **FAT Demon**. It can lead to spiritual fatness.

We cannot be spiritually fit until you do what God says to do; be obedient.

Prayers

I receive and use spiritual food properly. I reject spiritual **FAT**. I share willingly and gladly of my gifts and talents that the Lord has given to the glory of God.

I reject selfishness and self-centeredness.

I reject spiritual fat of any kind, in the Name of Jesus.

Physically Fat

We have discussed several kinds of spiritual fat, which is the collection of spiritual Bible-based information from any, and all sources, especially from your pastor. We've discussed Revelation Fat, Talent Fat, and Gift Fat. You have a spiritual gift and may even know what it is, but you don't move in it. That is not pleasing to God.

And now for the meat of this book, no pun intended, the physically fat, due to *spiritual causes*. People can be influenced by spiritual entities that drive them to eat. Every spiritual disorder that can lead to spiritual fat can also lead to physical fat.

The things that are seen are brought to manifestation by the things which are unseen.

The Bible tells us that the world we see is made by things which are unseen; the natural world that we see reflects the spiritual world that we don't see, (Hebrews 11:3). The food on your plate is not the only thing contributing to your size. When you become spiritually fat, which is invisible, then physical, visible fat can follow. What unseen things may be affecting you and your weight?

Candice left a church where she was flowing in ministry every Sunday and teaching her weekly Bible class for a church where she sits on the pew. She is collecting spiritually but not *giving* spiritually; that leads to spiritual fat. What is spiritual is translated into the physical; Candace has gained 20 pounds, (three dress sizes) in just a few months.

This is not a fat-person-bashing book, but it is a fat-bashing book. Anyone who is fat didn't just become fat overnight. Chances are something happened that changed either eating patterns, physical activity levels and patterns, or both. Those changes may have influenced metabolic rates, the way your body uses food, permanently or temporarily. That something that happened may have been spiritual or had spiritual or soulish consequences. You haven't stopped eating since so and so died. You never used to eat this much (or often) since the divorce. Your appetite picked up that summer you spent with relatives. Now you eat as much as Little Cousin Junior. Soulish and spiritual things, though unseen, affect physical things that are seen, even your weight and size.

Most people don't want to be fat, though some say they do. Kids proudly stick out their six-year-old stomachs after a big meal. But by the time they are preteen, most want to be slim to prepare to participate in the activities of teenage and early adult years.

Who wants you fat? God. No. The devil.

Let's weigh things out--, no pun intended. If you're physically running for your life, fat (or fatter) can mean slower moving and easier to catch. If the devil is shooting fiery darts at us (Ephesians 6:16), then our bodies must be targets. If a person is fat, then the target is easier to see. And hit.

If you are *spiritually* running for your life, then you are slower moving and easier to catch. You don't feel like praising or worshipping. You don't feel like praying. You're too tired to read the Scriptures or go to Bible study and don't even think about asking you to serve as an usher or in any church ministry. In that condition if the devil threw a spiritual problem at you, you'd fall apart. Physically or spiritually, you're at a disadvantage. You have got to make changes.

Physical Changes

Muscles appear on the guy that works out. The opposite will happen to the couch potato. Muscles will disappear on the person that doesn't exercise. Muscles burn the most energy in the body. If you don't have any muscles, you don't need as much food no matter how big you are. But folks with muscle can eat and eat but hardly gain weight, and they need to eat because that muscle is using up energy, burning calories. Eating will not make muscles, only making muscles and using muscles will make muscles. I am not necessarily talking about the bulky bodybuilder type, just well-toned, regular people type muscles.

On the outside and the inside, God has designed a remarkable body. It will change to reflect what you're doing with it. More aptly put, your body will reflect what you're doing to it.

Your body will change to reflect your lifestyle.

Spiritual muscles are also made by use. If you aren't using any spiritual energy, you don't need to receive any. This is how people dry up spiritually. They are not giving out anything to anyone else. They are not ministering what they've been given to anyone else. They may get fat for a while as they receive and receive spiritual food, but soon God will cut that off and they will dry up spiritually. This also happens physically. As long as you are using muscles they will prosper and be healthy, but when you don't, fat adds on and the muscles atrophy. They become weak and saggy from neglect and not using them.

Physiologic Changes

Eat enough chocolate, sweet cakes and bread and drink enough alcohol; the flesh will start to crave it. Remember when you hardly liked cola and now you drink it every day? Certain changes happen in the body to make you handle it. Some people drink a beer and get high off of it, but a single beer the next time won't have the same effect. The body creates special cells that use up the alcohol, so more alcohol is needed the next time to have the same effect. The same thing happens with caffeine, sugar, cola, and chocolate, this is not as obvious as with drugs and alcohol at first. This is how addictions begin.

Your body has certain cells that enjoy sugar, alcohol, and et cetera. As you eat more and more of the junk, the *I-like-junk* cells grow in numbers. Now there are twice as many, or four times as many junk cells. They want to eat, and they want **you** to feed them. They get more sugar, bread, cakes, and alcohol by creating a natural or flesh craving which creates the overgrowth which creates the craving which creates the overgrowths. It's a vicious cycle. The more junk cells, the stronger the craving is. It is a very real need to you. It will wake you up at night. It will keep you from sleeping unless you give in to it. Then it may calm down enough to let you go back to sleep. It will distract you at work. Cravings and addictions have no clocks. They don't care where you are or what you're

45

doing. Their job is to drive you, to give in to what they want you to do. **It's real, it's spiritual, but it's not God.**

Overindulging in sugars, breads and alcohol, for example, leads to an overgrowth of yeast in the body. This overgrowth of yeast causes chronic tiredness, mental dullness, dark circles around the eyes, and may contribute to allergies and other problems. If in great numbers, those bad cells may overrun normal, healthy cells in the body causing physical sickness, yeast infections, overgrowths are not always the kind advertised on the one- or three-day cures for on television, and they don't just affect women. Also, irregular eating can cause blood sugar surges, among other things. Too much of anything is a bad problem.

Declarations

I receive and use natural food properly. I reject unhealthy fat; I choose what I eat. It is not chosen for me. Food does not just happen. My body burns calories and fat efficiently. I'm not willing to lose anything else, but I am willing to get rid of weights and burdens in the natural and spiritual.

Recommended: *The Yeast Syndrome* by Doctor John Parks Trail Bridge, and Morton Walker DPM..

Disclaimer: If you don't exhibit any eating, snacking, or dining excesses, that doesn't mean you don't have any spiritual concerns. This book is mainly about the causes of overeating and the consequences of it, including fat. Do not misinterpret the fat demons to believe that God is giving you a clean bill of spiritual health if you don't find yourself in any of the preceding or following categories. This book is not suggesting that everyone has a problem. It outlines some problems. That may be caused by spiritual entities. Use Wisdom and the Holy Spirit to guide and confirm any spiritual diagnosis and reminders. Medically this book does not diagnose any physical ailments of metabolism or other function.

This book does not diagnose any emotional, psychological, or mental ailments. See physician were indicated.

This is a spiritual reference.

The FAT Demons

There are some *spirits* that influence and promote bad habits, such as drinking, smoking and drug abuse. And there are spirits that influence **eating;** I call them **FAT Demons**. They are sent to encourage overeating, eating the wrong foods, eating to distraction or obesity, to the end of not only not serving God, but by omission or lifestyle, serving the devil. If eating is or can be a temptation to you, then food is what the devil will use to tempt. If you're a Jack Sprat, you could eat no fat. Then the devil won't offer you food. But Jack had a wife who would eat no lean. That's who will be tempted by food and snacks.

People need deliverance from the spiritual oppression of putting things in their mouths, such as drugs, alcohol, and food. Babies and children try everything in their mouth. You've probably been told, ***Don't put that in your mouth,*** more times than you've been told anything else in your entire life. If you're still being told that about spiritual things, then you are not graduated from being a baby Christian. Don't put that in your mouth or, *Take that out of your mouth* is a parent's mantra. There must be a reason God wanted you to hear those words so often. Putting wrong things in the mouth is a temptation for too many, Christians included.

> **You've probably been told,**
>
> **Don't put that in your mouth,**
>
> **Or, Take that out of your mouth**
>
> **more times than**
>
> **you've been told anything else in your entire life.**

Food addiction is a reality. The demons and fallen angels' assignments are predictable. They are seeking to destroy God's work in the Earth with tested and tried spiritual weapons. You are not the first person to be tempted by food, excess, or sin. The assigned demon knows what you like and how to present it to you. A demon will not offer pork chops to Jack Sprat. **Where there is no desire, there is no temptation.** The demon's charge is to present something that will tempt, to bring disgrace to you and God's Kingdom if possible. We pray that it isn't.

Let me give you an idea of how much the devil hates you--, add up all the hateful, spiteful, hurtful things all the people you have known in your entire life have ever done to you. Satan hates you more than all of that hate added together because he put all of those people up to doing those things against you, and is still working against you.

Satan puts what's taboo in your path, and within your grasp, then tries to influence you to take it. If you're a thief, the opportunity to steal something you really want to steal will present itself. If you're an alcoholic, or drug user, he'll make those things available to you. If you are a food-*aholic*, then dinner is served. For Adam & Eve, it was forbidden fruit; what is it for you? What is your weakness? You don't have any; the devil can't get to you that easily... *you think?*

The devil will start with something that seems harmless, then try to move you to the sin where he really wants you. The *spirit of lust*, for example, begins with *vanity*. Oh, there's nothing wrong with caring about your appearance. But the *spirit of vanity* comes in, and is nurtured when you cater to it, by spending way too much time and money, and putting too much importance on how you look. Then *vanity* makes room for *lust*; don't you want others to notice how lovely you are? That's how it starts.

You've got to be spiritually alert at all times.

Other spiritual oppressions can start with food.

The Devil's got food for bait like a mouse trap, and you're the mouse. He's got things you like hoping to open the door to other distractions, dangers, and sin. The devil is trying to get your soul. What bait are you susceptible to? What are you likely to put in your mouth? Watch out for Devil hooks and mouse traps attached to that cheese.

Prayers

I bind and cast out every Snack Demon, Dining Demon, Eating Demon, every **FAT Demon**.

I bind up and cast out the *spirit of obesity,*

in the Name of Jesus.

I *loose* the *spirit of health and Wellness.*

I will obey my Momma, and finally take things out of my mouth that don't belong there.

I purpose to study, to show myself approved, and to be alert all times to the strategy of the enemy so I can be victorious, in the Nname of Jesus.

To the glory of God.

FAT Mouths and FAT Prophecy

Girl, if you don't stop eating, you're going to be big as a house. How many well-meaning relatives have spoken those words to you?

He's big boned like his daddy. You're going to be the size of a football player. How do **you** know?

How about these warnings? *You won't always be a size 8, just wait until you get a little older.*

Wait until your first baby. Wait until you're 30. Wait until you live a little longer. You'll see. Wait until gravity hits--, the midriff bulge, the love handles. You've got big feet. And you've got a big head. So the rest of you... You're going to be as big as a cow. Do I need to go on? **These are all words of the FAT Prophets.**

Who told them they could prophesy over you? Then why are you listening to them? Just because someone is older than you doesn't make them your personal prophet. They have no authority to speak into your life unless you allow it. Just because that "prophet" told you you'd be fat (even if it was your mother) doesn't mean you have to be fat. FAT Prophets are just regular people with a lot of opinions and loose jaws.

Who are these people who've been and are still telling you what size you're going to be? They are FAT Prophets, False Prophets.

There are countless thousands of people over 30 who still wear size 8, and thousands of women who have had babies who don't have pot bellies or love handles.

There are thousands over 40, 50 and older in size 10 or whatever size they choose. You do not have to gain weight just because you had a birthday. When a child is 5, he may wear a size 5, and size 10 when he's 10. That's the way it is with kids. But Lord, you don't have to wear size 40 just because you're 40. Ladies and gentlemen, you have dominion over your body. You can be any size you choose to be. The **FAT** Prophets are false prophets. They have lied and do lie.

What are you going to do about all the lies that have been spoken over you all of your life? As faith comes by hearing, (Romans 10:17), you should be hearing what thus saith the Lord instead of what thus saith Aunt Sally. She told you how many times what Mac and cheese is going to do to your thighs? You've also heard that you're going to keep eating it. For one, regarding the Mac and cheese, why are you still eating it? And two, why are you letting it do that to your thighs instead of not eating it or exercising, proving the FAT Prophets wrong? Are you trying to prove Aunt Sally, right? Then you can say my Aunt Sally is a prophet, she can tell who's going to be fat.

Fat Prophets are only speaking what they hear, what others have said over *them*, and what they may want to happen to you anyway. They can be right, you can be fat, or they can be wrong. You get to choose by *your* actions. Don't let the FAT Prophets' words dictate to you. And by the way, they told you some other wrong stuff too, but this book isn't about that.

Let's all let all that wrong stuff go. Release it to God. Ask Him if it's true. As for these prophets, they aren't being very spiritual if they were, they'd be saying what God says about you, not just reporting what they see with their natural eyes or what they think with their natural minds.

Huh? Are you your own FAT Prophet? Are you thinking fat thoughts about yourself? Are you racked with guilt about your weight? Are you increasing the weight of guilt you now carry by saying negative things about your weight, your size, your shape, or the way you look, in or out of clothes? What are you saying about your own desire or lack of desire and discipline to exercise? Are you talking to yourself and others about how fat you are? Then you are your own FAT Prophet. The devil has trained you well.

If I just walk past that dessert cart, I'll gain weight. Now you know that's not true. Is it funny? No. Can you find something else to make fun of? *If I smell food cooking it puts on pounds.* Is that true? No. Is it funny? No. Stop prophesying fat over your body and over yourself. You're operating the bad man-made principle of **fat comes by hearing.**

God says that faith comes by hearing, (Romans 10:17). What I'm talking about is talking about fat. Keep your mouth shut with a fat jokes and it'll be easier to keep it shut when the forkful of sweet potato pie or cheesecake comes dancing in front of your face.

You can be your own worst enemy, the world says. You can be your own FAT Prophet. Faith comes by hearing. How do you expect your body size and weight to decrease if you keep talking it up? Unless you are a liar and you don't even believe a word you say, think about it. Maybe you don't have anyone to blame it on, but you can change. Here's how:

- Stop making fat jokes about yourself. It is not making anybody like you more, especially your body.

- Stop saying what fat is going to pile on if you eat, go near or smell food; are you a comedian or a real person?

- Stop telling yourself how hungry you can get and bragging about how much you can eat a cow, a horse and ox, et cetera. It's not funny. You're not in grade school anymore.

- Stop making fun of your shape, your size, and any body parts that you don't like.

- Stop thinking any of these things about yourself in public or private. Cast down the thoughts before they become words, (2 Corinthians 10:5). If you don't know what to think, try Philippians 4:8.

- Stop squeezing yourself into things. Break free. Break free so you can *move*. Compressing fat keeps it fat. No one puts on a girdle to exercise.

At least if you're up and about. You're walking can benefit you somewhat. But if the muscles aren't moving, they won't be burning any calories or fat; break free.

Yes, I said, girdle--, if you're willing to be uncomfortable for hours at a time, try exercise. Don't wear your clothes so tight that you have discoloration and bruises on your skin. You've got to make some changes when underwires are hook closures are digging in and marking your skin.

- Stop trying to please others. If your spouse likes you heavy, but you want to be slimmer and fitter, you're going to have to please yourself. That's another whole book.

- Get to know yourself.

- Learn to like and love yourself in Christ.

- When feeling hungry, discern which are emotional soul cravings, which is a flesh craving and discipline yourself accordingly.

Don't be afraid to say I desire to be healthy and physically fit. Whatever that is to you, don't be afraid to say what you really want, even though it may sound funny the first time you hear yourself say it. Exercise your faith, then exercise your body. The Bible says we shall have whatsoever we say, (Mark 11:23). Don't be caught saying one thing at home then making fun of yourself in public. That's double mindedness bordering on self-hatred.

Your kids will think you're *loco*, then they will copy that self-defeating, self-deprecating behavior. You can be healthy and physically fit. If that's for you then claim it, speak it, then do what it takes to be it.

- Stop saying how you can't lose weight like you used to.

Metabolism doesn't necessarily have to decrease with age. Usually what changes is lifestyle, diet, and activity levels. Remember that you have dominion over your body, which includes how it works, how it moves, how it serves you, and everything else it does. Start telling your body what to do, and how to do it. **That's what the fat talk is doing, it is telling your body the opposite of what you really want.**

Have faith to say what you really want. Faith talk sounds like this: *My body works efficiently, and I burn calories and fat the way God intended,* or *I am healthy and physically fit.*

Don't give up. God is the Lord over all flesh, and that includes yours. And with God all things are possible. The Word says not to be led by the flesh. That is not just talking about emotions and soul cravings, it's talking about flesh cravings too. Do not let cravings and *I-wants* lead you. If you allow the Spirit to lead you, you will walk in temperance, self-control, health and fitness.

Come unto me all ye that labor and are heavy laden, and I will give you rest. Take my yoke upon you, and learn of me, for I am meek and the lion heart, and you shall find rest unto your souls. For my yoke is easy and my burden is light, Matthew 11:28-30

The Lord is inviting those who are heavy laden to come to Him. He will give rest, restoration to your souls. He further says that His yoke is easy, and His burden is light. That tells us that the burden of the enemy is not easy, it is difficult, nor is it light. Instead, it is heavy. That's how you know the difference between God's yoke and the devil's burdens. All that stuff you're trying to carry around is the devil's. All those emotions, all that hurt, all that guilt, shame, and depression is the Devil's. All that physical weight is the manifestation of the spiritual oppression. It is not God. It is of the devil. Come to Jesus and be restored to what God intends you to be.

Getting saved doesn't mean that all natural consequences of sins disappear. But if the sin never stops, the consequences never stop either. If you're already saved but going *through*, then be thankful that you have a relationship with God that gives you the victory and restores your soul. Be thankful that you have the Holy Spirit and use Him as the Comforter.

As faith comes by hearing, it's time you start hearing some right things. From whom? From yourself. For starters, the declarations and prayers provided in this book are good as a beginning. Use them to be your own prophet. Be a thin prophet, a slim prophet, a fit prophet, a health prophet over yourself.

Faith for good things comes by hearing good things. Faith comes by hearing. How many people have you prophesied skinniness to? And aren't they skinny? Remember when you couldn't gain an ounce no matter how much you ate? Wasn't there a Slim Prophet pronouncing that over you? Maybe the Slim Prophet was *you*? **Remember when you used to look in the mirror and tell yourself how good you looked?** What changed? Why did you stop? Are you waiting for someone else to do it? The words you hear were the first things that changed. The *spirits* that you allowed to influence you were the next things to change. Then your natural eating and exercise habits changed. Faith Comes by hearing. Skinny comes by *hearing*. Guard your ears. Decide what you want to hear from now on. It will affect what you become.

Prayers

I reject all false prophecy, the words that any FAT Prophet has spoken over me. I can have what I say. Therefore, I renounce all negative things I have ever spoken over my own body.

I will exercise my faith and my body.

I stop all negative talk and thinking toward myself and about myself.

I love myself in Christ.

I love myself.

I choose what size I want to be. It is not chosen for me.

I choose health and life.

I choose what I eat. It is not chosen for me.

I break free out of girdles and tight things so I can **move**.

The devil is bound and cast out, not me.

Excess weight is the devil's burden.

I am anointed of God. The Devil's burden is destroyed because of the anointing. I am anointed; therefore, I am free.

The Spirit of Obesity

FAT prophets can speak the *spirit of obesity* into people's lives. The *spirit of obesity* is made-up of the imps and entities that I call the **FAT Demons**. What do **FAT Demons** do and what does **FAT Demon** work look like?

People try and try to lose weight, but it doesn't seem to happen. There's a trend in families where everyone is heavy. But, when whole families live in the same house and have the same diet and exercise patterns, yet there are big differences between sizes we wonder what's behind what is seen. What is it that takes over a whole family for generations, or one member causing fat? Could it be a *spirit of obesity*? Yes, **FAT Demons**, the same that the fat prophets invoke with their words.

The *spirit of obesity* can be:

- Generational. Runs in families to 3rd and 4th generations.

- Transferred by contact, association, relationship, marriage.

- Influencing- Makes suggestions for the victim to follow.

- Oppressive- Weighed down by sin or the bondage of sin.

- Possessive- Resides with the person all the time. Incites ravenous cravings.

The *spirit of obesity* headed up by the *spirit or strongman of whoredoms* may have any number of little demons under it, which I have given easy to understand names such as the Dining Demons, Snack Demons, Chocolate Demons, Eating Demons, Coffee Demons, Ice Cream Demons--, named for whatever foods the devil may be trying to use to bring on obesity.

How do these demons influence or possess? They can't, unless you or someone you're related to, invites or lets them into your life. When your child begs for a cookie and you give in, that's the end of it, but a demon nags until you resist unequivocally, or give in. If you resist, that's not the end. That demon or another will try again. If you give in, that's the beginning. The relentless nature of spiritual attack puts you in a spiritual war zone. You've always wanted to be popular. You are. You are spiritually popular, like it or not.

Because demonic *spirits* travel together, if one is allowed in, it invites its cousins, which are like squatters looking for a place to dwell, the first demon who wants to visit or camp in your popular place, your body may be a Dining Demon. You and a lot of other Christians may judge a Dining Demon socially and spiritually acceptable. These demons are excused as, *Oh, she just has a big appetite*. Or, *You know, brother John. He's all man*. Or, *Girl, you really know food; you must be a gourmet*. These eating disorders are trivialized and made fun of. But once the demon gets in, it beckons for its cousins, which may or may not be socially or spiritually acceptable. His cousins. Smokers, Drug Users, Alcoholics, Adulterers, Sex Perverts, Gamblers and Murderers, et cetera. But the only way they can get in is if they are invited in by you or the open door that a lesser demon may have opened also with your permission.

Further, demons cannot be appeased or satisfied. They don't make deals, they just come to do what they've been instructed to do. Demons don't compromise. You can't reason with a demon when you give in thinking, I'll just do this one time. Nope, you just sprung the trap. The influencing or possessing demon isn't leaving after you indulge once. That's only the beginning. That's why there are generational *possessions*. They don't leave on their own. If they are not found out, put out, or kicked out, they will stay. They wait for folk to die and then influence, oppress, and possess their children into the same sin acts and bondages.

A good man leaves an inheritance to his children's children. A spiritually cursed man does the same thing, only it's not good. It's demonic.

When you think, *I'll just have one more then I won't ever do that again.* Don't deceive yourself. It may not be very easy to get over a bad habit or behavior. The influences of a demon may have graduated to an addiction and or spiritual possession by the time. By that time, if you don't care much about yourself, then think about your children, born and unborn, before you make the spiritual decisions that you are faced with.

It's easiest never to give in to demonic influence. It's easiest never to start a bad habit. Depending on your spiritual foundation and predisposition, resisting may not be that easy, but it is easier than getting over it. It's easier than suffering through it. It's easier than wasting time, money, and your life away--, until Deliverance. It's easiest for your children never to pass it on to them. It may not be easy to resist, but it is the easiest of all possible scenarios.

Don't give in to the **FAT Demons**. They don't leave readily, especially if you feed them. That means don't give in to their urgings, influence, and cravings. They don't die, they feed, they multiply, they try to increase their numbers, and then they try to cause you to increase in size. That is not the kind of multiplication you want. Resist the **FAT Demons.**

Prayers

I bind up and cast out the *spirit of obesity* and any work of the **FAT Demons** in my life and generationally in my family. I block and renounce every association with any friendship that gives place to **FAT Demons.** I *loose* the Spirit of God and the *spirit of health,* Wellness, and life, in the Name of Jesus.

The Dining Demon

Let's go out to dinner. Will you meet me for lunch? Let's grab a pizza Saturday night. A meal is always a good excuse for a date. Food is often the icebreaker to start a new relationship, good or bad. The *spirit of adultery* and the *spirit of fornication* both encourage eating. Their activities can center around eating or the pretense of eating. Worldly specialists say that if a mate's weight is mysteriously going up or down, watch for cheating. The person may be juggling another relationship that may revolve around meals, or they could be innocently losing or gaining weight. But sudden weight loss in a healthy individual could be the result of the *spirit of vanity.* or it could invite *vanity*. As said before, *vanity* invites lust. See how these oppressions work together?

The adultery or *fornicating spirit* is not sneaking food on the side, it is sneaking sex. It is working with its cousin, the Dining Demon, and using food as the cover up with horrible side effects and consequences. But it may have all started with a seemingly innocent dinner invitation. See how the devil uses something simple, adds it to something bad to cause something worse.

Foodwise, the Dining Demon has class. It eats in good restaurants. It knows what to order. It knows all the courses such as the appetizers, soup du jour, entree, and which fork or spoon to use at the right time. It knows the best cuts of meats, from prime rib to tomahawk steaks. This demon knows desserts. It is a *spirit* that influences or possesses by making folk believe they have *arrived* because of food and wine knowledge, style, etiquette and the ability to *afford* the lifestyle that goes with it.

This does not mean don't go out to dinner, but if you feel that you have overeaten and overspent every time you dine out, if you feel guilt or some other oppressive emotion, then there may be a spiritual component to this that you need to look into.

Maybe you've been told that you've have an eating disorder. Perhaps you do. Perhaps you don't. The problem may just be an influencing *spirit* causing the symptoms of overeating. Maybe it's a Dining Demon causing your voracious appetite, as you pursue the "good life."

Conversely, the Holy Spirit dwelling in you will cause you to exhibit discipline, moderation, self-control, and temperance.

The Snack Demon and Others

The Snack Demon is more of a blue-collar everyday demon. It influences the sneaking of food for eating in private. The Snack Demon will have you hiding food in secret places. Eating in the bathroom is not off limits to the Snack Demon--, is this disgusting or what?

Have you ever noticed how many very mostly heavy people aren't *seen* eating very much, but they maintain their weight? You've asked yourself, *when* are they eating? Well, they sneak food when no one is looking. I hope that's not a surprise to you.

God says don't overeat, but the Snack Demon and Chocolate Demons, and others are sent to encourage, convince, influence even possess the mind to do things against the express will and Word of God. One such possession is evidenced in the story of the pigs that drowned. The pigs had received 6000 demons that had been in one man, Legion. When the *spirits* entered the pigs, they ran off a cliff and drowned in the sea, (Mark 5:913). The demons wanted a human to live in. When they were in the man; they made that man crazy. When they entered the pigs, then the pigs committed suicide. *Sueycide.* Get it? (Pun intended.)

Hellish demons have been sent as emissaries of the Devil, and they want to dwell in you. They lead folks into temptation and sin because these demons have no body and they want to live. Over and over, life after life, they want to live and in so doing ruin lives, families, generations and bloodlines if they have their way, which is the way of darkness.

When a man sins, then the devil can say, *God, I told you so.* Satan is the Accuser of the Brethren, and the women*ren* and the children. Even if he is only accusing you of food abuse or overeating, but he desires worse sins of you.

Have you ever eaten and then wondered to yourself, *Why did I just eat that? I wasn't even hungry, and I didn't even really want that.* We're not going to say the devil made you do it. Perhaps there are things in your life that are influencing you, subconsciously. We'd all hope that we have 100% control over our lives, but do we? We should. The guilty voices of lying, FAT Prophets in your head, don't count. If you have weak or oppressive feelings after eating then suspect negative spiritual influence.

Eating for the sake of eating, not for nourishment, is a trick of the enemy. Advertisers make snacks look like entertainment. They want you to believe that movie plots are better if you're eating, ball games are more fun, et cetera, but none of that is true. After indulging, there may be discomfort or bloating after the pounds pile on. Misery, depression, feelings of being unattractive, among other emotions may compound the issues. Who remembers or cares about the plot of a movie or the score of the ball game after the problems from overeating show up such as fat irregularities, metabolism issues, or disease? Do you know why you set those snacks out in the first place? Do you have the habit of eating buttered popcorn when watching TV? Who taught you to do that? Do you want the food? No. Suspect the Snack Demon. The Snack Demon's job is to make you think you're hungry, not getting your share of food, or not satisfied. It's not cute, funny, nor is it something to brag about.

Check yourself. If you are hiding food or carrying it around in your purse, not for your children or for a medical condition, that may be a sign of food addiction or overeating in response to the influence of the *spirit of obesity's* Snack Demon. Food that is eaten in your car and places where no one is watching is *still* food and still has fat and calories. That which is done in darkness will surely be brought to light, especially sunlight--in that swimsuit at the beach.

Prayers

I bind and cast out every Snack Demon, Dining Demon, Eating Demon--, every FAT Demon.

I bind and cast out the *spirit of gluttony* and the *spirit of obesity* in my life in the name of Jesus.

I lose the Holy Spirit in the spirit of Wellness, health, physical vitality, and fitness.

I choose life.

The God of Health

Eating with the enemy.

Minister Erma Simpson, Basic Moves Ministry

When you sit down to eat with a ruler, consider carefully what is before you. And put a knife to your throat. If you are a man given to appetite, do not desire his dainties, for they are deceitful foods. (Proverbs 23:1-3).

Hunger Versus Appetite

Hunger is a God-given desire for man's physical survival. Hunger is triggered by the biological need for food. Most Americans have never experienced true hunger. The growling that we feel is the stomach letting us know that it is empty. Most times it is simply asking for water, not food.

Appetite is craving lust triggered by the sight, taste, smell or even thought of food. Appetite causes us to overindulge gluttony in food. And to desire foods that God is not recommended.

Note: Hunger may be satisfied while appetite persists after a meal. No man is hungry when he reaches for dessert. Many times appetite rather than hungry. Hunger causes us to desire and eat foods. That are not good for us.

Published with permission.

Whoredoms

Whoredoms (worldliness) is a *spirit --, a strongman.* Under its demonic umbrella is the lust for money, prostitution, adultery, fornication, idolatry, chronic dissatisfaction, excessive appetite and other things. *Whoredoms* drives the lusts for the feelings and experiences of the flesh life that lead to disaster, death and eternal damnation.

Idolatry

People hear the word *whoredoms* and may think of Hosea and his harlot wife, Gomer. But they will not think it has anything to do with them. Newsflash: *whoredoms* includes those who love to eat, idolaters and a lot of others.

When you say, *I just love Michael--* whomever *and he eats a certain breakfast cereal so that's what I'll have to eat,* that's idolatry. The world is filled with copycats. That's how most things are sold to people. Folks want to be like the Mikes of this world, and that's why celebrity endorsements work. Those stars and athletes may not even eat the food or use the product they advertise. If you're copying the image presented in TV ads, it's idolatry.

Or you might say, *I just love ice cream and I have to have it every day. I have to have my chocolate* or, *I need my coffee.* Perhaps you're saying these things to be conversational, mainstream, or clever. Do you really want to be identified by your *food*? Didn't your Mama call you pumpkin long enough? Wouldn't you rather be identified by the Name of Jesus? Do you want people to say, there she is, run, get her some coffee before she snaps? Or look, there's a woman of God. I wonder if she has a word from the Lord today.

Try this: *I love God. I've got to have God every day.* Pant after God. Crave God, worship God. We were not put here to worship food; that's idolatry. Some people say they live to eat. We should just eat to live. Amen.

Jesus tells us to have bread and wine and remembrance of Him at communion; that belongs to Jesus and no other. Pagan religions pay homage to false *gods* and to the dead by preparing special meals and pouring libations. If we are offering food and drink to any other than God, isn't that idolatry?

Prayers

I repent of not putting God first in all things in my life. I repent of worshipping, lusting after and or seeking anything ungodly in my life. I repent of not acknowledging God in my life's choices, even my daily life. God cares about everything

I do and everything I choose. I vow to seek God to direct my steps from now on. I bind up and cast out the *spirit of idolatry,* in the Name of Jesus. I *loose* temperance, self-control in my life. Deliver me, O Lord, in the Name of Jesus.

Excessive Appetite

Excessive appetite is caused by a *spirit*. God says that the man that is given to excessive appetite should take a knife to his own throat, (Proverbs 23:2) Suicide is not God's way, but is He saying that chronic overeating is suicide? Maybe. Probably. Excessive appetite is a spiritual problem for which deliverance is needed.

Relatives tried to avoid Ted's house on the way to the park because he'd eat their picnic lunches. Ted just ate and ate. Ted didn't inquire when people walked by with picnic baskets or really accept when offered food. Ted asked people sitting at his house, Did you pack a lunch? What did you bring? Insisting, he would cause car trunks to be unlocked and picnics foraged. If Ted saw food, he ate it. Sadly, he died a young man of about 350 pounds. Excessive appetite is a **FAT Demon**, and it can be a killer demon.

Eat Like a Bird

Some people believe they are hungry about every two hours, so they feed that hunger. Metabolically, it could be so--, hypoglycemia. People who are hungry every two hours usually eat like birds. Birds eat a lot. They eat little bits, often. That is actually good for you. The little bits are fruits, nuts, vegetables, and healthy foods that are quickly metabolized. These people are usually as thin as rails.

But many adults who take two-hour feedings are fat. They may have somehow confused the feeling of full with the confession of empty and set out to refill their stomachs. The full stomach may have been learned in childhood but is not optimum for human health.

But I'm Still Hungry

Yes, you are. With the deluge of processed foods on the market today and the depletion of soil nutrients in much of the farmland that grows the real vegetables we have to select from, many foods are lacking the very vitamins and minerals they're supposed to have. Even if you eat balanced meals, you may find yourself feeling as though you've missed something in your diet. Chances are that that something was missing from your food but eating more of that food may be too much food for your body. If you are one who experiences this, look into getting a non-synthetic) vitamin supplement to supply your body with the essential substances it needs, but continue to eat as balanced meals as possible. Limit the processed foods as much as you can, don't overstuff yourself because of a low nutritional value in the foods from which we must choose.

The stomach is not supposed to feel
full all the time.

Chronic Dissatisfaction

How often have you craved something but couldn't
exactly put your finger on what that something was?
A dill pickle could have been the beginning of an
eating bonanza, then a banana split, followed by a
pizza. You may have sent your spouse out late that
night for a burrito to top it all off. The next morning
you realize that none of those things hit the spot, so
you kept eating interesting things. A three-day eating
bench later, you finally admit that the flavor,
experience or sensation you sought never came in
contact with your taste buds.

Some of the dishes you ate came close, but they
weren't quite right, they weren't made right, too much
salt, not enough garlic, wrong sauce, nothing really
satisfied, but you ate so much of so many strange
things that you got tired of eating. You're starting to
feel guilty about overeating and simply stopped the
binge but did not get satisfaction.

Did you pray while in binge mode? What? Pray about
food? Yes, you do it all the time. You do it every time

you sit down to a meal, don't you? You pray that the food will be safe to eat, nourishing to your body. Some pray that it will taste good. **Why not also pray that the food will be satisfying to you?**

And the Lord shall guide thee continually, and satisfy thy soul in drought, and make fat thy bones, and thou shalt be like a watered garden, and like a spring of water, whose waters fail not. (Isaiah 58:11)

The world may suffer *chronic dissatisfaction*, it is spiritual and a part of *whoredoms*. The Rolling Stones sang, *I can't get no satisfaction* in the 1960s, but the very wise Solomon wrote about satisfaction first, even before Christ:

All the labor of man is for his mouth, and yet the appetite is not filled. (Ecclesiastes 6:7)

Man is ever working to fill his appetite, whether for food or material goods. Yet Solomon says it is never satisfied. The Israelites and their appetites were never sated. They were unhappy about the lack of water and food. They weren't pleased about the manna. They didn't like the Wilderness; what --, they liked slavery better? They complained about snakes. Considering all the livestock they had with them we don't even know what they said about the flies. Would you have complained? How many of you would have told God that you couldn't leave Egypt because of all the bugs in the Wilderness?

Don't answer that.

79

Sin Cannot Satisfy

As wise and rich as King Solomon was, even he wasn't satisfied. He acquired 700 wives. Those wives practiced idolatry and strange religions, which was the cause of Solomon's downfall.

As decadent and debased the lifestyles were in Sodom and Gomorrah, they still weren't satisfied. The men wanted to have sex with the angels God had sent to Lot. Why? **Because sin cannot satisfy**. That's why. You can't commit a sin and be done with it. It will leave you unsatisfied or dissatisfied. There was an old R&B song, *Do it till you're satisfied, Whatever it is, do it…* That can't happen since sin cannot satisfy. Worldly songs are always asking for one night with a certain person who is the object of another's desire. If not one night, the singer will ask for one illicit kiss or something else that seems almost innocent, thinking that one will be enough for them. But it's not. If you were ever to get that one opportunity and act on your desire, you'll be thinking on it, wondering about it, or maybe wishing or planning to do it another time just to *"get it out of your system."*

Doing it is what gets it **into** your system.

No matter how perverse, exotic, exciting, or whatever you want to call it, no matter how frequently you do it, sin cannot satisfy. This is why a Sinner falls into bondage repeating the SIN act over and over. Man may choose different partners, different settings, even different substances, but he can never get satisfaction from sin. There's not enough food to satisfy. There are not enough drugs. There is not enough sex.

Sin cannot satisfy, only God can satisfy.

I'm saved, and in the Body of Christ I expect satisfaction. God has promised it to me. If there's a *spirit of chronic dissatisfaction*, then there must be a *spirit of satisfaction*, the spirit that fills you when you get blessed by God. Every blessing from God, small or large, should be accompanied by this feeling. It's that *spirit of satisfaction* that I want every day. I ask to receive it, everyday, in the Name of Jesus.

I want my children to have the *spirit of satisfaction* so, they don't ask me to buy so many things in the stores, so they don't want to eat every time they see someone else with food. So, they don't throw down the toy they have in their hand and cry for their little playmates' toys.

I will abundantly bless her provision. I will satisfy her poor with bread. (Psalm 132:15)

God has promised to supply my needs (Philippines 4:19) to satisfy me with long life (Psalm 91:16) and

81

give me all things that pertain to life and godliness, (2 Peter 1:3). If a craving tries to come upon me, I recognize it may be the *spirit of dissatisfaction*, I will not give in to it. I will not let it in. I will not let it happen in my life. Instead of giving in to demonic suggestion, I must open my mouth and resist, speaking the Word.

Satisfaction is a gift from God, the Gifts of God are not, for Satan and his Kingdom. If a demon has been in existence for 2000 years, for example, and has influenced 30 lives, and maybe possessed at one time or another 10 and all those people have eaten all the ice cream they could get into their mouths, and the demon still isn't satisfied, it will never be satisfied. (Hell and the
grave are never satisfied, (Proverbs 27:20.)

Prayers

I bind and cast out every Snack Demon, Dining Demon, Eating Demon, every FAT Demon in the name of Jesus.

I *loose* the Spirit of God, Wellness, health and wholeness in my life.

God has promised me long life and satisfaction.

I am satisfied in Him.

I will finally obey my mother; I will not put things in my mouth that shouldn't be there.

I do not put things in my system that are not therapeutic or things I do not want there permanently.

My system is clear of sin by the Blood of Jesus.

spirit of addiction

What's the difference between a chocolate addiction, a drug addiction, and a sex addiction? They are all addictions. Addictions do not please God. The devil may want to introduce addictions to you in subtle and likable ways. He may start with food. A food addiction might start with a simple family tradition, then move into a bondage. You can't have Thanksgiving without sweet potato pie. Then it may move into addiction: that pie was so good, we need to have it every holiday, then every Sunday. You get the picture.

Maybe you say you **don't** have a food addiction. What is your food history? You may make a banana pudding, for example if you will eat the whole thing, then don't make it. Every time you see chocolate on the menu, you've gotta order it. I tell you in love, you've got a problem. A food connection for anything more than nourishment and sustenance of the body is dangerous because the devil may try to start with food and add or substitute other things to entice or entrap you.

For example, many people who smoke didn't pick up the first cigarette, planning to develop a habit or an addiction. Many smoke after eating, or in some cases, instead of eating. Addictions can start so innocently, but ruin and take lives. Look in the ICU Intensive Care Unit of any hospital and see the patients dying because of devastating lifelong addictions and many of those addictions were food or food related.

As it relates to dieting, where's the Wisdom in creating the habit of consuming chocolate diet milkshakes instead of a meal for several days or weeks to lose weight? It seems that a craving for chocolate flavored milkshakes will result, and if you give in to it, the weight will be quickly put back on. How do you shake that habit?

Desire for food can start as a craving, then persist into addiction. To justify addictions, obsessions, poor eating, laziness, and bad behavior people say you have to die of something. If you read your Bible, you'll learn that you don't have to die sick. You can get called away because it's your time. Psalm 91 says with long life I will satisfy him. That means I can live as long as I want to and healthy at that. I can live until I'm satisfied, and that is what I'm going to do. You could get raptured. You don't have to die of an illness or disease, accident or disaster. But we have to choose to live. Sin is death and righteousness is life; I **choose** to live. You must make your choice too. Choose life, (Deuteronomy, 30:19)

**I don't have to die of anything, to the
glory of God.**

Food addictions, if they don't kill, they become the forerunners of addictions such as sex, drugs, and alcohol. Are they the tricycles of the more dangerous addictions, which are the bicycles and motorcycles? Could be. I don't know as well as you do. Has your food or other addiction gotten worse or better over the years? You can tell if you are becoming addicted to more or fewer foods than when the addiction first began, and if the frequency of usage has increased or decreased. Have other addictions been added? Don't you think it's time to break the *spirit of addiction* that's running or ruining your life? Use the Name of Jesus, because of the Name of Jesus, every knee will bow, (Philippians 2:10)

Addictions can go away all at once with God's deliverance and strong resistance or taper off with discipline. I've heard people say, *I used to love pizza and now just can't stand it*. The addiction either went away or into remission or was replaced with something.

Addiction remission? Sure. Maybe your addiction isn't active right now. You've seen people put down cigarettes for weeks, months, or years and then suddenly picked them up again. That was addiction remission as a trick of the enemy, where the demon that influences the addiction doesn't rage like it once did. It may even hide. You may have prayed and believed God for deliverance, and it appears that you have been set free, but you may not really have deliverance as long as you are not giving into the demons' urges. Your health may be intact, but don't risk letting it take over again. Don't risk passing it on to your kids; get rid of it. You may need strong intercession and spiritual deliverance.

A remission may be apparent if you conquered the addiction in the flesh, but not in your soul and spirit. That means you made-up in your mind to quit. You decided to quit smoking, for example, but nothing happened in your soul or spirit life. So that spiritual influence, fleshly need, or soul craving that drove you to begin smoking in the first place still exists. You've just decided to ignore it. How long do you think you can do that? Or you may have already replaced smoking with something else, like eating.

Why should you care about the spiritual reasons for overeating? Because you don't want to just lose the weight, you want to get rid of weight and burdens and you wanna keep it off. If you lose the weight instead of getting rid of it along with what caused it in the first place, then you may find it again. Jesus' rebirth and renewal must happen spiritually since it is a spiritual battle. You can only be sure of that when it is bound up at the roots and cast out in the name of Jesus.

Prayers

I bind up and cast out the *spirit of addiction,* in the Name of Jesus.

I *loose*, Temperance, self-control and spiritual deliverance, in the Name of Jesus.

I am not willing to lose anything else in this life, but I am willing to get rid of excess weights and burdens.

Spirits of Fear and Worry

As mentioned, the *spirit of fear* can be a **FAT** Demon. It can freeze people in their tracks in the natural. It can keep someone in the house when they could be outside. Exercising outside is where members of the fellowship take walks. It is where the church plays volleyball. Fear puts on many different faces. Fear of people and their faces is spoken of many times in the Bible. There could be a fear of playing in the game. Dropping the ball or losing the game, the fear of letting others down. That's why God says not to be afraid of their faces. Don't be afraid of any of the faces of fear.

The *spirit of fear* can immobilize. It keeps people seated when they should get up. It may keep you from walking in the morning around the school tracks. Are you afraid of the neighborhood dogs, cats, or bugs? You may think that you're not going to lose any weight anyway? That's the fear of failing.

The *spirit of fear* can bring on a case of nerves and anxiousness that may cause eating. Some seek comfort food like chocolate, breads, pasta and desserts or complete junk food buffet eating everything in sight. This may lead to the hand-to-mouth disease of raising food with one hand to the mouth and eating mindlessly. This eating may accompany other mindless activities such as watching TV. The *spirit of fear* can add pounds; it is a **FAT Demon**.

Or maybe you don't overeat because of fear, but fear can freeze the digestive process. Some know it is heartburn, gas, or reflux. Others know it as butterflies or knots in the stomach. When you're afraid, the blood that is supposed to rush to the stomach to digest the nutritious food you've just eaten is rushing to the extremities, in a fight or flight response. Fear sends blood to the arms and legs, for running away or fighting. This is why people who have nervous stomachs don't eat before public or major events. This is why people who get anxious speaking to crowds probably shouldn't eat before giving a speech. Depending on how gripping and chronic the *spirit of fear* is, it may mess up metabolism in a worse way than just gas or indigestion. Fear may permanently cause improper digestion and irregular bowel elimination. Improper bowel elimination can cause worse problems than fat.

The *spirit of fear* may have come from your mother as an infant. She overfed you, both too much and too often. She stuffed you because she was afraid you were not getting enough to eat, and now you're used to being what I call stomach-conscious--, you can't sleep without it. That infantile overfeeding increased your brown fat cells, which predisposed you to being heavier in adulthood than you might otherwise be. The *spirit of fear* is of **FAT Demon.**

Fear causes missed opportunities, lost jobs, careers and ministry. Then because of it, on a secondary level, feelings of uselessness, defeat, self-loathing, and unforgiveness may flood in. All of this, unchecked, can lead to depression. Fear is a **FAT Demon** that can open the door for other **FAT Demons** such as the *spirit of depression.*

Worry

While eating, the mind is on the taste buds. After eating sufficiently, you become stomach conscious. All the while you're not thinking of your outside problem, are you? Have you noticed people who hum, sing or wiggle their legs while eating? They have forgotten the cares of this world. Food has become an escape and a distraction for them. As mentioned earlier, eating can be a very real distraction. Always be spiritually alert. Worry and escapism are only distractions, and they are **FAT Demons**. When you get through eating, the same problems will still be there. But if your weight increases because of the eating, then there are added problems.

Phobias

Fear is no small thing, and the devil really isn't playing with you. Little phobias should be overcome and cast out as soon as you are aware of them. No longer should you announce *I'm afraid of...* anything that is a foothold for the *spirit of fear* you need to overcome. Fears of everything from spiders to snakes to cats to dogs, monsters, thunderstorms, dentists, whatever. God has not given us a *spirit of fear*, but of love power and a sound mind, (2 Timothy 1:7). If you have the fear, you don't have the other three. **Would you rather have one bad spirit or three good ones?**

You might be saying, *It's just a little phobia.* Good. It's an opportunity to work your little faith. The world tells you to accept yourself with all your faults and weaknesses. But a phobia isn't part of you. Fear didn't come from God, so you must reject it. It is a foothold for the devil, a trick of the enemy, and this is war.

God says to cast down imaginations. He says, **Fear not**. Over and over again in the Scriptures He says **I am with you.**

The first line of defense is resistance, but you have even greater weapons against the devil than he does against you. But don't forget, the devil is a spirit, so you've got to use spiritual weapons.

Prayers

I bind up and cast out the *spirit of fear*, in the Name of Jesus.

I loose the spirit of love power and a sound mind.

I purpose to conquer every phobia, in the Name of Jesus to the glory of God.

I resist the devil, and he flees from me.

I untie eating from worry, fear, and phobias.

Anger, Unforgiveness, and Bitterness

Unbelievers, or uncommitted Christians, seek payback on the person with whom they're angry. Living well is the best revenge. But many people, women especially, go to the kitchen for a carton of Haagen Daz or Ben and Jerry's to plot revenge.

How many people have you heard say, *"I was eating everything in sight, and then the answer came to me"?* None. No one. It's like the people who look up in the ceiling for answers to questions--, they are not there. When you eat, blood goes to the stomach for digestion. In order to think and plan, even if it's revenge strategy (not recommending it, unless it's against the devil), because blood needs to go to your brain, not to your stomach for digestion. **Food cannot answer anger. There are no emotional answers in food.**

Your Mama taught you how to eat, *right*? Maybe you have a strange desire to get back at her or prove yourself grown up by eating all the things she told you not to eat as a child.

Ed didn't like sharing with his sister, so now he eats an entire large bag of snack chips and one sitting just because he *can*. This started out as a way to fill a deficit he's felt for the past 35 years. Whether emotional, (did Ed feel unloved, jealous of his sister), or fleshy (was he still hungry)? He doesn't know, but now the flesh is taken over. He's addicted to snack chips.

It is dangerous when the emotions drive the flesh. Emotion-driven flesh can influence anything from overeating to crimes of passion, at the very least the *spirits of anger, unforgiveness* and *bitterness* are **FAT Demons.**

Did you get to that? I'm telling you that if you **forgive** so and so, even the horrible things that he or she did to you, that you can **lose weight**. The pain in the heart of the past episodes in your life is a weight in the spiritual and soulish realms. It may also be the cause of weight that is manifested in your physical body. It is a burden. Forgive, stop hating. Put away the bitterness. Let those things go and watch the weight go with it. You must get rid of these fat demons. They are. Clinging onto you by your emotional hopes.

Prayers

Vengeance is the Lord's.

I don't need to claim revenge except to follow the Word of God. And be active spiritually in warfare. I don't need to eat when I am angry.

I untie eating from anger.

I put away the works of the flesh, such as anger and pride.

Pride

The *spirit of pride* could be a **FAT Demon**. Many fat people, especially those who have socialization problems, are overly prideful. They want to be right all the time, even if it means proving others wrong. It's a 24-hour a day thing for them. If they can prove another person wrong, they themselves won't look so bad, *they think.* These people eat. They are inundated with the *spirit of pride* and *obesity.*

They are inclosed in their own fat, with their mouths they speak proudly. Psalm 17:10

God did not make a mistake in describing these people as being enclosed in their own fat. Literally. They are so full of pride and self-righteousness that there is no room for anything else in their lives. They are so prideful that they cannot even forgive *themselves* for making mistakes, so they don't make any. At least that is what they want to believe--, and have you believe. They are so emotionally wounded inside for feeling as though they are less than perfect for past and unconfessed mistakes that they believe are hidden. They are unforgiving of themselves and others, so they eat and eat when no one is looking.

Maybe you are not engrossed in your own pride yet. Maybe you're just a little prideful. You may be calling it perfection. Maybe you mean well and don't want to do anything wrong. Perhaps you just get a little angry when people accuse you of having done things incorrectly. Perhaps it's a soul deficit where your mom or dad constantly criticized you when you were a kid.

As a child, maybe your schoolteacher criticized you, even publicly embarrassed you. Now you want to prove them all wrong by being perfect. Maybe you crave praise, but when you can't get it, you may resent others or try to discredit those who are very successful or get a lot of attention and appreciation. Pride is a **FAT Demon.**

If you are a child of an alcoholic parent, you may have a real perfection problem. You could be running over with pride. Don't be embarrassed. The confession of pride can be a private act, entirely between you and God. Confession is the start to get rid of pride--, this **FAT Dining Demon**.

Prayers

I untie my emotions from food. I untie eating from feelings of pride. I put away the works of the flesh, such as anger and pride.

Spirits of Shame, Guilt, Self-Pity

Any of the sins that make you want to hide or hide some aspect of yourself physically, emotionally or spiritually potentially bring **FAT Demons** activity with it. **I wonder if Adam and Eve gained weight after sinning.**

Guilt, shame, fear, self-pity and **depression** are

Hiding Sins. If you're under the oppression of one of these emotions, then you may be influenced by a **FAT Demon.**

Dee picked up the staff lunch one day. The office splurged on burgers and fries. By the time the food got there, everyone was very hungry because it was after 2:00 PM, so they started eating like lumberjacks. Dee nibbled her lunch, feeling all eyes on her although none were. She suddenly blurted out, *"I already had a combo in the car. I didn't want you to see how hungry I was."* Dee was having twice as much food as everyone else, but we all thought she was eating the same or less. Dee was hiding food and being heavy. She was hiding her true self. The *spirits of guilt* and the *spirit of gluttony* are **FAT Demons.**

Shame is a **FAT Demon**. Some people have endured a horrible past and don't want to be attractive on purpose. With the help of their Eating Demon, because of shame, they'll cover up the beauty that God intended them to have. They think they are hiding behind their heaviness. Usually these are such pretty and attractive looking people anyway. They have a beautiful presence and good hearts. They will find themselves attracting people anyhow, but not feeling comfortable doing so.

That light that God put in you cannot be hid. Even though there are **FAT Demons** trying to help you hide and enclose what God put in you, it cannot be hid. Get back **FAT Demon**, ministry is coming forth and the child of God will be happy, healthy, and comfortable too.

Prayers

I untie my emotions from food.

I untie eating from feelings of shame, guilt and other emotions that make me want to hide.

I put away the works of the flesh. Such as anger and pride, guilt, shame and fear.

I put on the Holy Spirit of God with power, love and a sound mind with forgiveness and self-control.

Spirit of Infirmity

Not everyone who is infirm, or sick is heavy or fat. Some small people are sick because they can't gain weight. We are not talking about them in this book. The reason I called the *spirit of infirmity* a FAT Demon is because of the sympathy sick folk get.

When children don't feel well, adults feed them. Kids get candy, snacks, and favorite foods to cheer them up. If food can cheer you up, and we all ought to be pleased as punch right about now. Children often get a burst of energy after eating. They may want to get down from the table and dance around and run and play. That energy surges from the increase in blood sugar levels, not from being *food happy*. I've never had a food to make me happy. Energized, yes, but not happy. Ask any depressed person what food makes them undepressed, and they will tell you, *"None."* Counseling is their medicine, and God has prayer and deliverance for depression, not food.

Sympathy feedings could fatten up a patient. Then the patient is miserable and other emotions may flare up. Don't overfeed yourself or your child in the attempt to be *cheered up*.

Alcohol toast also boasts the word, *cheers*. Alcohol is a mood elevator first, then a mood depressor. Alcohol can really put on the pounds; it's a **FAT Demon**, too. They can't cheer you up any more than food can. A lot of the time the food that you enjoy and have been eating is what has made you sick in the first place. Food can be a weapon of the devil's warfare.

Another way the *spirit of infirmity* may cause weight gain is the secondary effect of prescription medicines. Steroids, for example, can really cause quick and dramatic increases in size. Marge, a petite young woman, was a size 4 at the beginning of summer. Suddenly she was a size 16 at the end of the same summer. And she was only 4' 9."

A lot of medicines cause discomfort, so you may be eating just to settle or avoid stomach cramps. Some drugs and medicines make you feel hungry. Then eating is to satisfy real or perceived hunger.

The Bible calls drugs, sorcery. Those drugs that are mind altering are more dangerous during the time the drug is working. You may become more susceptible to demonic influences when the drug wears off. Suddenly you're hungry.

I am not telling you to put down any life- preserving or life-improving drugs. Consult your own physician. Just know what your physical and spiritual concerns will be from using certain drugs.

* And. Obviously, some infirmities affect your ability to move around and exercise, adding to fat.

Prayers

I don't have to die of anything.

I bind up and cast out the *spirit of infirmity*.

I *loose* the Spirit of God, the spirit of Wellness, health, and wholeness in my life.

I use drugs therapeutically under wise counsel of physicians, Dr. Jesus and the Holy Spirit.

I leave no room for spiritual influence that is not of God.

Spirit of Divination, Sorcery

Drugs (sorceries) may increase appetite. Even therapeutic drugs (prescriptions that promote healing) sometimes increase appetites, especially prescriptions with the label: Take With Food. A habit of taking medicine with food, or food with medicine when you might not need to, just to be sure, is a way drugs bring on weight. This is especially true of long-term drug therapy. The tradition of, mom did it this way, or sick people get all the ice cream they want may pile on extra pounds.

Recreational drugs can cause incredible cravings and many people consider it a joke to munch or binge after using certain drugs, especially marijuana, maybe while intoxicated or high out of control of the mind. Control of the mind and the body affecting and gain temporary control and strongly influenced the user.

People can crave foods after getting over a drug, alcohol or cigarette addiction. One can get over an addiction, but the *spirit of addiction* can persist. When Martin, who is unmarried, became saved, he gave up fornication and adultery, which he admits he used previously for entertainment. He gave up sex for God, but now he eats at least two pints of ice cream a day to make up for it. These sugar rushes make Martin silly and giggly, and give him the sense of feeling happy. He is using this particular food as a drug. The body's not designed for extreme sugar rushes, such as the kind that comes from sweets and desserts. This is dangerous to his system. Martin traded a sex addiction for food addiction. It's the same spirit, different substance. Remember when you used to love ice cream sandwiches, than a certain candy bar, and replaced that with another food? Food can become very addictive. What's more it's legal, it doesn't cost too much, and it's easy to score.

Warning: Replacement addictions aren't always food. For food, as in Martin's case, a sex addiction was replaced with food. The converse could occur. A food addiction could be replaced with a sex addiction. Or something worse. Don't allow it. Take charge of your body, mind, and soul so you can be used in the Kingdom of God.

Maybe food was never a temptation for you until you got over a certain habit--, say drugs or cigarettes. If so, you've gotten over the habit, but not the addiction. You still have work to do. You still need physical and spiritual deliverance.

**If abused food can be a mind
and body altering drug.**

Prayers

I bind up and cast out all the works of the devil in my life.

I bind up and cast out the works of drugs and sorceries.

I use drugs therapeutically under wise counsel of physicians, Dr Jesus and the Holy Spirit.

I'll leave no room for spiritual influence that is not of God.

Spirit of Heaviness, Depression

Got the munchies again? What will it be this time? Depends on what's bothering you, doesn't it? If you're feeling depressed, you might want something to cheer you up, like chocolate. If you're feeling happy, you might want something to celebrate and have some chocolate. If you're feeling sad about a relationship breaking up, you might want something that will make you feel better, maybe some chocolate. If you're mourning the loss of a loved one, you might want some real food, like mom used to make, some soul food. You might want to finish that meal up with some cake. Maybe some chocolate cake. Sounds like you got a Chocolate Demon and it's not cute, funny, nor is it something to brag about.

You've heard folks say it. Gotta have my chocolate.

Who's gotta have it? You or the demon?

The Chocolate Demon is not the only eating demon. Many of these other demons eat and encourage aggressive appetites to oppression. It's the flesh response spoken of earlier soul cravings. Maybe chocolate made you feel better the last time you went through this or something similar. Maybe Mom always gave you cocoa when you were unhappy or not feeling well.

Depression can lead to heaviness. You don't think God named it *heaviness* by mistake, do you? Heaviness is over-grieving where the normal grieving period might be six months or a year, or person who is under the bondage of the *spirit of heaviness* might still be grieving for 5 or 20 years later. They may have grieved their life away as a perpetual victim, widow, or divorcee. Heaviness is much worse and escalated than depression. Both can lead to acute and chronic eating, especially if you are conditioned to reach for that *happy food* to fix the blues you feel.

Recommended my book, **Seasons of Grief**,

Prayers

I untie eating from feelings of sadness, disappointment and depression.

I bind and cast out all the works of the enemy in my life, depression, heaviness and sorcery, in the Name of Jesus.

I *loose* the Spirit of love, power and a sound mind, in the Name of Jesus.

The I Don't Care spirit (Apathy)

The *I-don't-care spirit* is part of the *spirit of depression*. Don't ever say that you don't care what happens to you, even if you really don't care. By speaking that it opens up a big wide gate that lets in all kinds of demonic oppression. Even if you feel like you don't care today, don't say it. Because tomorrow, prayerfully, you may not feel that way. Hold your peace.

A living body is very attractive to a *spirit* that's looking for a place to dwell. The spirit has its assignment and its own agenda, which is **against** you and the natural. If you knew someone didn't like you, was against you, or was out to get you, would you invite them to stay in your home? No. Would you tell them they could come if they wanted to? That you didn't care if they came or not? No. But that's what you're doing spiritually when you say you don't care. Now, in the spiritual, you've got to make the same decision and declarations as you were in the natural, or you could get any kind of spiritual houseguests.

By saying you don't care, you risk being overtaken spiritually. That's why the Word says that you were either hot or cold; the lukewarm *I-don't-care* spirit can be run over.

Milk that sits out becomes lukewarm and all kinds of bacteria and germs can grow in it. If drank it can make a person sick. That same sour milk has all sorts of life in it that you can't see, but if you take it into your body. It can cause big health problems. There are unseen *spirits* that may try to influence you if you don't state what you will and won't allow.

Just as in the world, if you don't vote, the candidate will be chosen for you. The same applies in the spiritual. If you don't choose a side, one will be chosen for you. If you don't choose God, the devil will send whatever he can get into your life. Rebuke the *spirit of I-don't-care*. Spiritual ambivalence is an open door to the devil. Be hot or cold, but do not be lukewarm.

Do not ever say you don't care what happens to you, even if you feel that you really don't care.

Regarding physical ambivalence, have you ever thought about what size you'd like to be? Seriously, do you care or are you just doing whatever, eating whatever and letting nature take its course? Do you feel that you have any control of your body, or your life? Ambivalence and *I don't care* will create *whatever*. Decision will create what you want, something really close to it, or something even better. Why don't you decide what you really want?

Then speak that.

Prayers

I reject the *spirit of apathy* in my life. I care what
happens to me. I care about my spirit, mind, body
and soul. I choose what I eat; it is not chosen for me.

I choose what size I want to
be; it is not chosen for me.
I choose God.

I choose the Holy Spirit.

I choose life.

Slothful Spirit

Maybe you're just plain lazy. You don't want to get
up in the mornings. You don't want to exercise. You
want to take a nap. As soon as you eat. Something
could be wrong with you, or there may not be
anything at all wrong with you. The *spirit of
slothfulness* could be enjoying sleeping your life
away for you. Get up. This *slothful spirit* is a **Fat
Demon**.

Hair Bondage

Maybe you have a legitimate cause or excuse for not exercising--, your hair. This one defied a category. Hair bondage is not a type of weave, or maybe it is. Maybe it's idolatry, vanity, or a real bondage. It depends on why a person acts the way they do because of their hair. This is cultural, so if you don't understand, ask someone.

Those in hair bondage don't exercise or don't exercise regularly because of elaborate and often expensive hairdos. I struggled with this one myself. Whether to fully exert oneself in regular exercise or preserve the $80, $200, sometimes $300 hairdo was the question. Did I want to look physically good and wear ponytails so I could exercise, or did I want to look coiffed, taking my chances on what my body physique would become as it reflected my leisurely lifestyle.

The Bible says that we should not be vain or overly adorn ourselves. Our beauty comes from the inside and it comes from within. The Bible says that the bodily exercise profits little compared to spiritual gain. Is that license to not physically exercise? No.

Folks in earlier days didn't have aerobics because just to eat and live, they worked on farms. Because they worked so hard, they didn't need exercise gyms. Our grandparents and parents could eat more foods than we can today because of their lifestyle. They needed more food to fuel all the labor-intensive farm work they did. We don't need that same food. We don't need that same food or that same amount of food to go to the grocery store, or order from a restaurant menu, then sit down and watch a movie. If you're going to eat like a farmhand, then you've gotta work like a farm hand.

Balance is the challenge.

Eating farm style food while living in the city style lifestyle will lead to fat.

Prayers

I reject the *spirit of laziness.*

I thank God my body moves. And move it with purpose to keep it healthy and bring it under control.

I will eat the kind of amount of food that correlates to my lifestyle.

I bind up and cast out the *spirit of ignorance*, the spirit of not knowing what to eat, when to eat, and how much to eat.

I *loose* the Spirit of Wisdom in feeding and caring for my own body.

Spirit of Procrastination

Maybe you're not lazy, maybe you're just gonna do it later or tomorrow. Exercise. Eat right. Go to church. Put that idea on the market. Tomorrow will be a better day. After all, it would be easier tomorrow. There is a right timing and a right season for everything in the economy of God. But false is the idea that the better time is tomorrow. God says now. Faith is (Hebrews 11:1), so everything is not best done later. The *spirit of procrastination* is a **FAT Demon.**

Prayers

I reject the spirit of procrastination.

Now faith is, therefore, I will do it now.

When the Lord says move, I will move.

The Late-Night Demon

The late-night demon is under dishonorable mention. Go to bed. Staying up late at night does more harm than good. It robs you of valuable and needed sleep and rest. It robs you of productivity the next day. It affects your appearance, especially as you mature. Look at all those dark circles or wrinkles around your eyes? Go to sleep.

While you're awake, what are you doing?

114

Anything important? You're probably watching TV and thinking about what you're gonna eat next. Cupcake. Soda. Coffee loaded with cream and sugar? The late-night demon is a **FAT Demon.**

Your momma's been telling you and now I'm telling you, go to sleep. Take that out of your mouth and go to sleep!

God spoke to many in dreams in the Bible. God can finally talk to you when you're quiet and sleeping. Go to sleep. You may be missing out on some spiritual guidance and direction. Go to sleep. I pray many times and go to sleep to wake up refreshed and with the answer to my prayers. Go to sleep.

The body is supposed to fast food for several hours. That's why the morning meal is a break-*fast*. This is designed by God. Don't violate it. Go to bed. Overnight or oversleep when your body is still, things are quiet in the natural and fasting. It's like your cell phone, overnight it is plugged in an connected to WiFi—it gets backed up. Overnight when you are plugged in to God…

Stop trying to act like a grown up and **be** a grown up and go to sleep. Discipline yourself with proper rest. Follow the laws, the natural laws of God.

It is vain for you to rise up early and set up late, for so he giveth his beloved sleep. (Psalms 127:2)

115

Declarations

I will get my rest.

I will fast several consecutive hours a day.

Oversleep 8 hours is recommended.

I will be quiet to hear what the Lord has to say to me. 1
Thessalonians 4:11

The Crowd Demon

Everyone else is doing it is not reason enough to
start to do anything. Everyone else was drinking
coffee in college between classes. At first I didn't
know where everyone went when we had a break, but
then I, too, found the coffee room.

I was not raised with coffee in the house and never
tried to drink it, yet I could *pay* for a cup of coffee,
that I didn't even want and pretend to drink it just to
be where the crowd was, just to socialize. Wrong
reasons, wrong *environment*, wrong people to make
friends with. But in my late teens, I didn't know that.
After a while I started drinking coffee--, *sort of.* The
same applies with food, cigarettes, and any other bad
habit. You may now be eating some stuff now that you
really never wanted to start eating, you've got to resist
peer pressure.

116

Because everyone else is doing it is probably more of a reason not to do something than to do it.

Jesus talked differently to the multitude than He did to His disciples than He did to his favorites. Do you want to behave like the crowd, as the multitude does, or are you strong enough to stand out when it means no one else is doing what's right? The Crowd Demon is a **FAT Demon.**

Good 'N Fat

Many folks think that fat is better, especially in babies, so they overeat and overfeed their children. Yes, fat babies are cute, but not necessarily healthier.

Know that there are some good things in fat. There are good fats that you should eat. Some help your cholesterol, for example. Some fats are essential. That means your body can't make them, so you've gotta eat them in your diet. There's good in fat. Antibodies are in fat. Antibodies help your body fight illnesses such as colds, viruses, and bacteria. People who are too thin can find themselves sickly, sneezy and ill more than nonskinny people, so some fat is good. There should always be a balance. Experts report What is ideal based on special measurements and tests?

The challenge is balance.

Being heavier than you should could cause your heart to overwork, among other adverse reactions. Carl died at the age of 30 of heart problems. He weighed nearly 500 pounds. The average man weighs 170 pounds. Carl was the size of three men. The heart works based on how. Which blood it has to pump and how much to how much body? His heart worked more than three times as much as it would have if he had weighed 170. So at age 30, he had overworked a heart. That could have hypothetically rested him to each 90 or coral cause of death might read heart abuse.

Balance is crucial. The challenge is balance.

Prayers

I reject false balance. It is an abomination to God.

I proclaim balance in my life. Both physical, financial, emotional. Everything that should be balanced is balanced, in the Name of Jesus.

The Skinny & Fat of It

Spiritual bulimia occurs when eating up the word, then rejecting it or not applying it for whatever reasons. Maybe the person next to you on the Pew made you mad. The pastor's wife had on another new suit and hat. Maybe you're already angry at your husband when you got to church. Blame it on anyone you want. God says that the Word falls among thorns, (Mark 4:7), but it is rejected, and no fruit comes of it because of the cares and distractions of the world. A person who may hear the Word and reject it is as the spiritual bulimic and the spiritual anorexic. Anorexic, frail, weak and undernourished.

The above are two examples of spiritual disorders such as binge eating--, bulimia and anorexia can cause metabolic disorders. Isn't this world we live in strange? Every kind of fattening substance you can think of is offered then you are told that you need to be thin. Go figure.

Prayers

A false balance is abomination to the Lord.

But a just weight is his delight. Proverbs 11:1

I will delight in the Lord as I balance every part of my life. Physical, spiritual, emotional, financial, and social.

I can do all things through Christ, which strengthens me.

The Discipline of Not Being Fat

At the Feast of Life all manner of sumptuous fair is presented to you. You're to use Wisdom and discipline in eating. God told Adam and Eve not to eat of the tree. The devil came in with the very first advertising campaign--, an informercial. We don't know how long it took him to convince them, but we know he presents the same tree that's been standing there all along. He highlights the fruit, tells them what it will do for them. He talks about how it's going to improve them and make them better than they already are. Like what? God didn't do it right the first time? Ever since the fall of man, the devil's been suggesting the menu, even for Christians.

Lust of the flesh, lust of the eye, pride of life (1 John 2:16). The Devil is using the same tricks. Why do you think that restaurants *display* the food they want you to order? Why do you think they have dessert cards and dessert trays? Why don't they just tell you about the sweets they? Don't just tell you about the sweets anymore. They bring it to you and let your eyes lust after it. It's the same little trick.

There must be discipline. That's what defines a disciple. All manner of spiritual things are being offered to you, as well as natural things. IYou know which spiritual things to choose, don't you? You also know which natural things to choose. Start with the discipline of food, the discipline of eating, the discipline of not being fat. It is something everyone can do, Romans 12 says it's your reasonable service. God knows you can do it, and he expects you to. He expects you to present your body a living sacrifice, holy and acceptable. God knows where. God knows there are temptations in the flesh life. James tells us that he does not give us greater temptations that we can bear. I believe. God.

Paul says he keeps his body under (1 Corinthians 9:27). *Under what?* Under control of his spirit, which is under the influence of God's Spirit. The man who walks by the Spirit does not fulfill the lust of the flesh. The lust of the flesh is what is pricked by **FAT Demons** to stimulate the appetite and cause the men of God to overeat.

The devil wants to take you out.

If that means out to dinner first, he'll do it.

Overeating may shorten the lifespan, lessen your ability to travel for evangelism, or impair your testimony. Perhaps you have the heart for dancing in your church's dance ministry. But you're out of condition. How does that glorify God? He knows your heart. Yes, he does. He knows that is overworked from that extra weight you've been toting around. An extra 5 pounds of weight, for example, requires an additional mile of blood vessels.

To be excellent Disciples of Christ, we can start with the discipline of food. Let's bless the Lord, and ourselves in our eating habits.

Then there's the Ministry of the discipline of not being fat. What is that? As a teacher, preacher, counselor, evangelist, et cetera, you will tell and show people what to do and how to live their lives. As a Christian, you represent God. Don't embarrass Christians by misrepresenting. Are you practicing what you preach or are you not preaching some things because you don't live it out? Have you limited your ministry because of your *lifestyle*? If you do not have and appear to have control over your own life, situations, body, et cetera, how will people receive you? How's your credibility? What will they perceive as your ability to guide, teach, direct, and exhort them.

The discipline of not being fat has a ministry of its own and that same discipline will tremendously enhance your credibility and ministry.

Prayers

As I am a disciple of Christ, spiritually I am a mind disciple. I want the mind of Christ.

I am a disciple in my soul. He restores my soul.

Physically, I bring my body under control. My body and my appearance speak to people before I ever do. Before and after I ever do.

I am a delight to the Lord in balance. False balance is not for me anymore.

My body changes to reflect my godly lifestyle.

My lifestyle changes to reflect my true commitment to God.

Prayer & Fasting

Some only come out by prayer and fasting. That's why you starve a cold. If you don't feed a cold, it will end faster. Take in clear liquids and plenty of juices--, similar to the same things you would consume in a basic fast and the cold will come out. Stay away from heavy foods and dairy products such as milk and cream products. They produce mucus, which is what you're trying to get rid of. God has cleverly inserted an involuntary fast in with the common cold. What the devil meant for harm-, his nasty germs and viruses God has turned it for your good (Genesis 50:20). You can be cleaned out in the process of having cold.

God has cleverly inserted an involuntary fast in with the common cold.

Some only come out by prayer and fasting, (Mark 9:29), *spirits of addictions* flee quickly with fasting. Cigarette smokers, drinkers, lust and drug addicts have reports of good success when fasting food and the addictive substance.

Is not this fast that I've chosen to loose the bands of wickedness and undo the heavy burdens and to let the oppressed go free. And that you break every yoke, Isaiah 58:6

Some of the main *spirits* that come out by fasting are the ones that influence eating. If you don't feed a stray cat, it won't stay at your house. If a Dining or Snack Demon tries to influence you to eat and you don't give into it, it will leave even if you have given into the Chocolate, Ice Cream, Soda or Snack Demon in the past. If you start resisting now, it will flee from you. If you don't think you can go cold turkey with all the snacks and foods, then resist the demons one at a time. Try resisting or fasting the Soda Demon for a week, then a month, then several months. Conquer it, then moved to the Chocolate Demon. You can do it.

I personally fasted chocolate for a full year to prove to myself that I didn't love it more than I loved God. Now I can take it, leave it.

Submit yourselves, therefore, to God. Resist the devil, and he will flee from you, (James 4:7).

The first time you resist will be the hardest. It may be something like withdrawal from drugs, alcohol or cigarettes. You may get real physical symptoms such as shaking, nervousness, jitters, anxiety, crankiness or irritability, but you can do it.

Think about your victory over food, what it will do for the rest of your Christian walk. Think about your testimony. Think about what it will do for your witness and your ministry.

- If you can resist this demon, think of all the others that will flee along with it. They like to travel in packs.

- Generationally. Look at what it'll do for your family. You won't be passing fat demons to your children.

- Think about the discipline you will achieve for your next victory. God will be taking you to the next level. Glory.

You're resisting the **FAT Demons** because you want to be obedient to God and resist the devil. You want to be an overcomer, not an overeater. If you're doing it for vain reasons, to be cute, to wear little outfits to entice a man or woman, it won't work. You must have the right motive in the right heart. By not eating, you may actually lose weight. But the list of your spiritual advantages may not be attained.

Prayers

I resist **FAT Demons**.

127

I fast to cause them to flee, to the glory of God.

I break all generational curses in my family.
Especially those in regarding food.

In the name of Jesus.

Spiritual Stream-lining

God chooses foolish things to confound the wise. Water is used to put out a fire, yet water can burn fat. Huh? Elijah built an altar for the sacrifice of bullocks against the prophets of Baal. Elijah's altar had the sacrificial fat **and** was doused with water, but it burned anyhow, (1Kings 18:33-38). That's God.

That's a spiritual point. In the natural water is necessary to burn fat. If you were to study the biochemistry of the body, which we won't do here, you will find that water is necessary to breakdown fat into energy. This is why water will help get rid of fat.

Prayer

I think and I drink--, Water.

Excess weight--, the Devil's burden is destroyed because of the anointing.

I am anointed.

My body changes to reflect my godly and anointed lifestyle.

Water

Water is mentioned in all 66 Books of the Bible. If you inspired holy men to write a Bible, why would you have them talking about water all through it? There must be something to water.

And God said, let there be a firmament in the midst of the waters, and let it divide the waters from the waters.

And God made the firmament and divided the waters which were under the firmament from the waters which were above the firmament. And it was so Genesis 1:6-7

God separated the waters above from the waters below the firmament. Above and below the heavens -- there are waters in Heaven.

Praise him you waters above the heavens.

Psalm 148:4

And he showed me a pure river of water and life. Clear as crystal, proceeding out of the throne of God and of the lamb. Revelations 22: 1

This didn't make a lot of sense initially, but since there was so much talk of water in the Bible, I knew it was important. Water is used in a number of different applications in our everyday lives or is used for baptism, which is a covenant. So God continues to confound the wise by using something that can dissolve things as a sort of glue that binds. (Matthew 3:11, Mark 1:8, 10; Luke 3:16, John 1:26, 31,33; John 3:5. 3:23; Acts 1:5). Only God!

Water is used to wash with to cleanse our external self --, our skin (Matthew 27:24, Luke 7:44, John 1:3-5). It is said that when impurities and sicknesses sweat out of your pores, you should wash them away as soon as possible to prevent them from going back in through those same pores by simple osmosis. You'll be healthier if you keep your external body clean, and you'll keep more friends. Doesn't it stand to reason that you can be healthier if you keep your insides clean too? (Quote from Minister Erma Simpson, Basic Moves Ministry.)

There's also prosperity in water. Remember the fish with the coin in its mouth? (Matthew 17:27). God has put so much in water.

Water is used in and for healing in the Bible. (John 5:34, 21). When water was walked on in Matthew 14:28-29 Jesus asserted and demonstrated His Sovereignty; He was as waters from above, walking on waters below. Jesus, our Supermodel showed that we have dominion over everything, including *the waters below,* earthly powers and even powers beneath the *waters below.*

Water is a beverage or drink in the Bible, (Matthew 10:42. Mark 9:41, Luke 16:24, John 27: 9; John 4:7, 4:10, 13:15, John 4:46). Why would God have the Prophets and Apostles report something as mundane as the drinking of water?

God is not mundane, and He is not trivial.

The voice of the Lord is upon the waters. The God of glory thundered. The Lord is upon many waters.

Psalm 29:3

God revealed what waters above and waters below meant. Water is spoken of in the Bible many times as *power*. (John 7:38, John 4:7-15, John 19:34) and water is power in the natural; hydropower turns water wheels, propels boats, helps make electricity and other things. Spiritually, there are waters above in the heavenlies--, God and His heavenly host.

But there are waters below, Satan and his fallen angels. The waters above have power and dominion over the waters below. When you as a saint drink common water it becomes those waters above because the greater one is in you, (1 John 4:4). The waters above walk over the waters below.

Drinking water, as in fasting, flushes your system. Fasting drives out demonic influence or oppression. Drinking common water washes out those **FAT Demons** that want you to drink sodas and eat junk all day. They will flee.

132

The Bible tells the story of a man sentenced to hell, who wanted one drop of water, (Luke 16:24). He was in a dry place where there was no water. This dry place was devoid of the spiritual water that we know that flows from the throne of God. This man thirsted and longed to be cooled. Yet because of his sins, there was no water for him, not one drop.

Camels are the only animal species that can store water for another day. We have to drink natural water as we need it while we can. We have to take in all the spiritual and living water we can while we can, so we will not end up in a dry place with no water. The evil spirits of the devil are ravenous and scavenger like. They look for dry places to land, dry places to rest.

When the unclean spirit is gone out of a man, he walketh through dry places, seeking rest and finding men. Matthew 12:43

Biblically, a dry place is where there is no Living Water, where there is no Spirit of God. It is where there is no Word. An evil *spirit* cannot dwell in the house where the Spirit of God dwells. Notice I said *dwells,* not influence. A Spirit-filled Christian can still be tempted, influenced, and still make some unwise decisions. If you are an occasional churchgoer, only read your Bible on Sunday--, a few verses at a time during the sermon with the rest of the congregation, you don't have much Word in you. You're pretty dry. You can be tempted and influenced when tested. You can fail. Dining demon, Snack demons, and other Fat demons can come in, among others if they choose. You don't have much to resist them.

If you want to resist the devil, then fill yourself daily with living water. Then drink plenty of natural water... And share.

And out of your belly shall flow rivers of living water.

For whosoever shall give you a cup of water to drink in my name, because you belong to Christ early, I say unto you, he shall not lose his reward. Mark 9:41

I used to think Mark 9:41 meant that God wants us to be nice to people--, offer them a cool drink if they're thirsty. If you're a person that God needs to tell to be nice, then be nice. But people are thirsty for the Word of God, for the Good News of Jesus Christ. That is the cup of water that you offer them. Great will be your reward in Heaven when you minister to those you meet.

Jesus told the woman at the well that if she knew who He was, she would have asked for Living Water. (John 4:10)

People know you're Christian and someone ask you for Living Water. What will you offer them when someone is hurting? Needing peace, restoration, healing, and hope spoken over them, what will you offer?

Will you be in a hiding place thinking about yourself and your trouble with **FAT Demons**, or will you be there for them? That's a devil strategy to have you sitting around all day, being:

- Stomach conscious. How do I feel? What do I want?

- Thinking about your weight.

- Thinking about your size or appearance.

- Thinking about your social, financial, marital, personal situations.

- It will make you.

  o Depressed.

  o Static. No ministry can come out of you.

That's enough. It's time to come out of that place and be what God has called you to be. Resist that devil and he will flee from you, and you will be free to minister your testimony and the Word to those who have a need-, in season.

Be victorious over **FAT Demons,** and bring forth ministry.

> **For you know the grace of our Lord Jesus Christ, that though he was rich. Yet for your sakes he became poor, that ye for his poverty might be rich. 2 Corinthians 8:19**

In the above passage Jesus became poor. *In what?* Money? Goods what? What is the last thing Jesus said before He said, **"It is finished"?** He said, **"I thirst,"** (John 19:28). Our Savior hung on the Cross, bearing all the sins of mankind. God could not look on Jesus in that state and turned His back on Him. Jesus became sin so that we would be sent free. His heavenly Father could not look on Him because He became poor in Spirit. He was without the Spirit, without power, he said, **"I thirst."** What did He thirst for? Not natural water. He had fasted 40 days to prove He could do without natural bread and water, but He yearned for Living Water.

God, our Father, heavenly water. Waters above.

> **Ho, everyone that thirsteth come to you to the water, and he that hath no money come, ye buy and eat.**

People, it's free. God is offering and offering. You keep praying and praying, asking God --, what is the problem? *Lord, help me. Lord, deliver me. Lord, bless me.* All through the Scriptures God kept sending people to **water** for restoration, for baptism, for drinking, for healing, for prosperity, for life, for thirst, spiritual Living Water is free, and He keeps offering it over and over.

Won't you accept it?

And he said unto me, it is done. I am alpha and Omega, the beginning and the end I will give unto him that is a thirst of the fountain of the water of life freely. Revelations 21:6

DRINK WATER

Why do you think God is offering us so much water? Because there's life in it. It's so simple. A thing that we need every day, a thing that is so commonplace that all we have to do is to drink. And it will bless us so much it becomes what we need it to become. Take it and drink it. In underprivileged countries or societies are oppressed, among the first things to go are potable water, and freedom to practice their faith; ever thought about that? You've got both! Ever thought about that?

Water is Deliverance. Pharaoh's army got drowned. In what, soda pop? No water. God led His people out of Egypt, a type of the world. Even though the Wizards had powers and the gods of Egypt had powers, it could not match the power of God. In their exodus, God parted the waters. He separated the waters. Of the powers of the world from the waters of the powers of heaven, God is in control. God is control of the waters, and He has given you Dominion. He has shown you how to have dominion over waters below.

The FAT Demons will persist if you don't drink water, the FAT Demons will take over if you don't take authority. Drown them, drown them, drown all the devil's little **FAT** Army just like Pharaohs army got drowned.

Water is power. Did you know that a man is more than 70% water? You are more than 70% **POWER**. You are really full of what you need to live. So then shouldn't you be living a victorious life?

Prayers

God is sending me to the water. Water has everything I need. Health healing, sight quenching. Life coolness cleansing.

I think, and I drink water.

The spiritual and the natural kind.

I'm Melting…

When water got on the Wicked Witch of the West in the Wizard of Oz, she melted. When water gets on your fat cells as though they melt. Every time you drink water, think of the **FAT Demon** work you are destroying. Water is used in and as deliverance over and over in the Bible. Let water be your deliverance from fat and the **FAT Demons.**

Drink and think.

Drink water.

Drink and think.

Maturing women seem to gain more weight than men. It could be that they don't drink as much water as men. Ladies, just because you're grown up, that doesn't mean you should drink all the cute stuff you served at your childhood tea parties. The cute drinks and the pretty stemmed glasses with the umbrellas, flowers and garnishes don't help you. They hurt you.

Accept God's offer to go to the water.

Drink water.

Rebuking the Devourers

Bring me all the tithes into the storehouse, that there may be meat in my house, and prove me now herewith, saith the Lord of host, if I will not open the windows of heaven and pour you out blessings, and I will repeat the desire for your sakes. Save the Lord of host.
Malachi 3:10-11

It's so simple. **Don't have the blues when you've got the clues.** God says that he will rebuke the devours for us. The Dining Demons, the **FAT Demons--,** they devour, and they cause you to devour. Snack, Chocolate, Ice Cream, Buttered Popcorn, and Cola Demons may all part of the Devourers. Or, you may be your own devourer! In the sense of eating and weight, you may be devouring your own cash. Answer This simple question:

What do you spend your money on?

- Food.

- Clothes.

As the sizes change, the wardrobe must. Larger clothes cost more money, (more fabric). Are you paying more for your clothes than average size folk? You are your own devourer.

Take back what the devil has stolen from you. Do you have a closet full of clothes that don't get you? Hundreds, maybe several thousands of dollars of clothes that you are *going to get back into?* Fight for your stuff, get in shape and wear your clothes, that the devil has stolen from you. Some people actually have two and three of the same item in their closets and different sizes so when their weight changes, they think no one will notice. A friend will notice, but a stranger won't care.

- Shoes.
  - I bet you just love a nice-looking pair of pumps or slingbacks. But the more weight you put on those shoes, the quicker you'll wear them out. If you have to keep buying shoes because of weight, you are your own devourer.
  - Fad diets and pills.
  - Exercise programs, equipment, and supplies.

Go to the **cause** and stop messing around with the symptoms. Why are you eating, spiritually? Remember that which is unseen brings into manifestation that which is seen. Are you doing it on purpose? What things can you do that you haven't tried yet? Have you addressed the spiritual nature of your life?

After all, you are spirit.

Drink and think.

Drink water.

Drink and think.

God says He will rebuke the devourer for our sakes, and He will pour out blessings from Heaven, (Malachi 3:10-11). What is He pouring? Waters from above? He's pouring out **Power**--, Power to handle the situation, Power to deal with things, Power to trample over the enemy. Power to bind up and cast out the enemy. Power to get the things that pertain to life and godliness and keep them. God is pouring out life-giving water, refreshing water from the Throne of God--, both spiritual and natural water. God is showering us with heavenly Authority, Dominion, power, and blessings to use as we need.

What does money have to do with this? God says you must be faithful in the little things and He will handle the big things. Really, no pun intended. God will rebuke those **FAT Demons** for your sake, in the Name of Jesus.

- O Are you Saved and in the family of God? Are you water baptized in Jesus' Name?
- O Are you Spirit-filled and flowing with rivers of Living Water?
- O Are you faithful in your tithes and offerings?
- O Are you faithful with spiritual knowledge you've acquired? And do you choose to acquire more spiritual knowledge? Or do you just want to know enough to *get by* in life?
- O Are you faithful with the spiritual revelation that God blesses you with, including gifts of the Holy Spirit?
- O Are you faithful with the natural gifts, talents, skills, and abilities that God has blessed you with?
- O Do you do in the natural as much as you can? Then you're ready for the prayer.

Declarations

I pay my tithes to the Most High God.

I give offerings fit for a king.

God rebukes the devourer for me.

I do not waste money on food, clothes, fads, diets, exercise equipment or plans.
When it comes to buying anything, I am wise, and Spirit-led

Recommended. Don't Refuse Me, Lord 4-part series. By this author also **When the Devourer Is Rebuked,** mini book.

Bind & "Lose"

Maybe you haven't cast the **FAT Demons** out because you didn't know they existed, or that you had any, or that you needed to, or that you could. Maybe you were too embarrassed to ask anyone. It's a new day. Let's bind and *loose*. **FAT Demon** warfare, shall I say, bind and **lose**? (Pun intended.)

Father, my Creator, Savior, and Redeemer, You are the Lord of the universe. You are the Lord of my life. I bless Your name. Your name is excellent in all the Earth. The whole Earth is filled with Your glory.

Father, if I'm spiritually fat, I repent right now, in the Name of Jesus. If I have received spiritual information over the years let me share it by ministering to others in need and season.

Father, forgive me if I have revelation that You have imparted to me to release, according to Your Spirit, that I have not released yet. I repent, and I ask for Your forgiveness.

I repent of not moving, not speaking when given a Word of Wisdom, or a Word of Knowledge, or a Prophetic Word, tongues or interpretation.

Lord, I repent, in the Name of Jesus if I have sat on the Pew with gifts, talents, skills, and abilities while my church has gone without, I'm sorry and I declare this day that I will no longer be a bench warmer when you've called me to be first-string.

If I've rejected Your Word after having heard it as a spiritual bulimic because of offenses or the cares of this world, Father, I repent in the name of Jesus. If I have not sat under the Word enough to receive proper proportion as an anorexic, I repent, in the Name of Jesus, and I commit to being a good Christian and right standing with You.

You said in Your Word that if we confess our sins that You are faithful and just to forgive and cleanse me of iniquity. Thank You, Lord, for forgiving me and cleansing me.

Father, in the Name of Jesus, I put away all works of the flesh: Pride, anger, bitterness, idolatry, unforgiveness, shame, selfishness, guilt. I put away all the works of the flesh, and instead proclaim that I will walk after the Spirit of God.

Where spiritual fat may have clung to me, I release it, I repent of it. I remove it now, in the Name of Jesus. Any eating disorder, eating proclivity that is associated with any of these spiritual influences, I rebuke and release also, in the Name of Jesus.

Where physical fat may have manifested in or on my body, I reject it; I bind it up and cast it out, in the Name of Jesus. I keep only the fat that is good.

You said in Your Word, (Matthew 18:18) that whatever we bind on Earth will be bound in Heaven, and whatsoever we *loose* on Earth will be *loosed* in Heaven. Father, in the Name of Jesus, I bind up and cast out any spiritual influence that has affected my appetite, whether it be idolatry, excessive appetite, chronic dissatisfaction, pride, anger, guilt, shame, depression, heaviness, infirmity, soul cravings, and natural cravings, excessive appetite for bad food, junk food, sweets, snacks, stimulants or anything ungodly.

I bind and cast out *whoredoms*, sex sins, lust and perversion, in the Name of Jesus. I bind and cast out *fear, selfishness,* or any other emotional demonic oppression. I bind and cast out sorceries, in the Name of Jesus. I bind up and cast out and reject the words of all Fat Prophets over my life. I renounce any negative words that I've spoken over myself and my body.

I *loose,* in the Name of Jesus Christ, the Holy Spirit, the *spirit of peace,* a *spirit of reconciliation*, and soul restoration. Satisfaction. Health, and balance in my body. I release the *spirits of selflessness,* and *self-esteem,* . **forgiveness, love, power**, and a **sound mind**.

I *loose* what You say about me, Lord, in the Name of Jesus, I thank You. I bless Your name, Lord, as health and spiritual righteous and rightness manifest in my life. I give You all the glory, honor and praise, Amen.

Declaration

Get back FAT Demons, ministry is coming forth in the Name of Jesus.

Special thanks to:

Basic Moves Ministry, Minister Erma Simpson.

Evangelist   Bonnie   Chambers
Doretha Harris, Super Duper sister

Other books by this author

AK: The Adventures of the Agape Kid

AMONG SOME THIEVES

Blindsided, Has the Old Man Bewitched You?

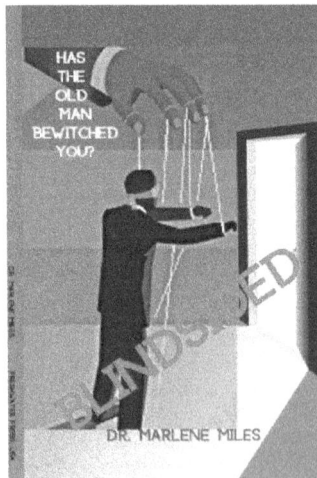

Churchzilla, *the Wanna-Be, Supposed-to-be Bride of Christ*

Demons Hate Questions

The Devil Loves Trauma

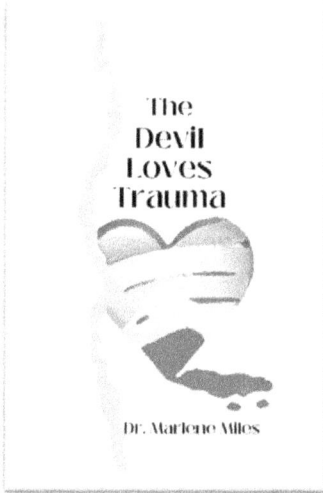

The
Devil
Loves
Trauma

Dr. Marlene Miles

Don't Refuse Me, Lord (4 book series)
Don't Say That to Me every apple
The FAT Demons

The Fold (4 book series)

    The Fold (Book 1)

      Name Your Seed (Book 2)

The Poor Attitudes of Money (Book 4)
Do Not Orphan Your Seed got
HEALING? Verses for Life got LOVE? Verses for
Life got money?
How to Dental Assist

Let Me Have A Dollar's Worth
Man Safari, *The*

Marriage Ed. *Rules of Engagement & Marriage*

Made Perfect in Love

Power Money: Nine Times the Tithe

The Power of Wealth *(forthcoming)*

Seasons of Grief

Seasons of War *(forthcoming)*

The Spirit of Poverty *(forthcoming)*

Warfare Prayer Against Poverty

When the Devourer is Rebuked

Wilderness Romance, *The (3-book series)*
        *The Social Wilderness, The Sexual
Wilderness , The Spiritual Wilderness*

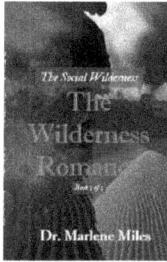

Journals & Devotionals by this author:

The Cool of the Day – Journal for times spent with God

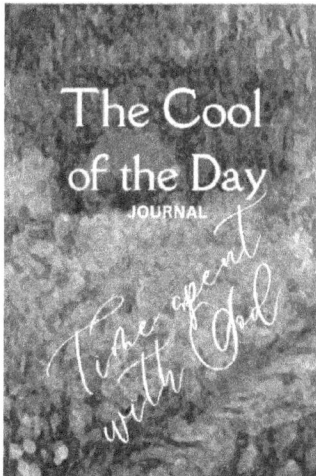

got LOVE? Verses for Life

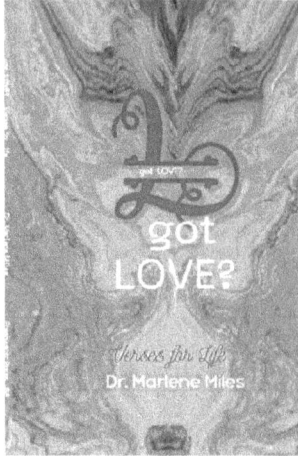

got Joy? Verses for Life
got Peace? Verses for Life
He Hears Us, Prayer Journal in 4 different colors

I Have A Star, Dream Journal kids, teen, young adult & up.

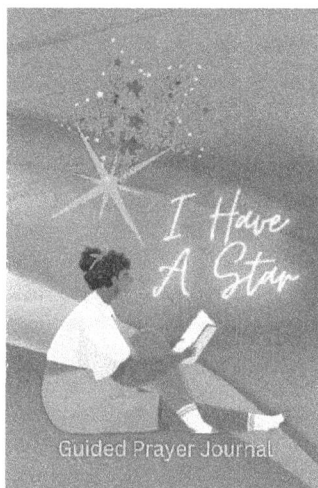

I Have A Star, Guided Prayer Journal, 2 styles: Boy or Girl J'ai une Etoile, Journal des Reves

Let Her Dream, Dream Journal, multiple colors

Men Shall Dream, Dream Journal, (blue or black)

My Favorite Prayers (multiple covers)

My Sowing Journal (in three different colors)

Tengo una Estrella, Diario de Sueños